Philosophy for Medicine
Applications in a clinical context

Edited by

Martyn Evans

Pekka Louhiala

and

Raimo Puustinen

RADCLIFFE MEDICAL PRESS
Oxford • San Francisco

Radcliffe Medical Press Ltd
18 Marcham Road
Abingdon
Oxon OX14 1AA
United Kingdom

www.radcliffe-oxford.com
The Radcliffe Medical Press electronic catalogue and online ordering facility.
Direct sales to anywhere in the world.

British Library Cataloguing in Publication Data

A catalogue record for this book is available from the British Library.

ISBN 1 85775 943 5

Typeset by Acorn Bookwork Ltd, Salisbury, Wiltshire
Printed and bound by TJ International Ltd, Padstow, Cornwall

Contents

Preface

'The unexamined life is not worth living', said Socrates. This is a rather uncompromising statement. But, if it is often true of life in general, it seems likely to be true of many particular lives and of many particular kinds of lives. The particular lives that we have in mind in this book include the clinical lives of doctors and other healthcare professionals, lives which revolve around a concern to understand the obstacles of *other* particular lives, presented to them by their patients. The doctor obviously cannot leave their patients' lives unexamined. Examining patients is the doctor's central task, and (if we leave aside self-limiting or otherwise trivial illness) a life which is unexamined *clinically* may find itself in danger of not being worth living or even, in extreme cases, capable of being lived at all. But neither can the doctor leave her own life unexamined, in terms of understanding, coming to grips with, reflecting on the daily challenges that her work brings to her understanding of herself, her professional role, her objectives and her aspirations. Moreover, the doctor cannot leave *life itself* unexamined – for modern technological medicine forces us to reflect closely upon what constitutes life as such, and upon how it is shaped both generally and individually by the circumstances which befall us as patients.

This book is meant to be an introduction to the habit of examining life in the philosophical sense which Socrates had in mind. It is an introduction to the philosophical questions which inevitably arise in medical practice in all its forms, and in the conceptions of human life (and of individual human lives) which inform medical theory. In producing this book, we want to bring to the attention of medical practitioners – and of patients, and of anyone interested in medicine's gaze upon the modern human condition – the questions which philosophy raises about human nature and about the way it is engaged by medical practice. These questions range from the reliability and applicability of medical knowledge, through the roles of ethics, aesthetics and spirituality, to the way in which our experience of the world is dominated by our bodily form and nature – be that experience a normal or a pathological one.

The book came about when a group of teachers and students of philosophy of medicine decided to give up the labels that differentiated them (as teachers or students, as philosophers or medical doctors), and to work together to try to get a deeper understanding of the practice of medicine. So it was that, following a very engaging seminar deep in the mid-Wales countryside in 2001, the three editors of this book agreed that enquirers from small countries like Wales and Finland could ask large questions about the near-global practice of biomedicine, with the help of their friends – primarily from Wales and Finland, but also from countries as distant and diverse as South Korea and the United States. Happily, our publishers – Radcliffe Medical Press – agreed, and this book is the result. We hope that you will enjoy it, but we hope still more that you will find that the examined medical life is, for patients and doctors alike, one that is well worth living, and worth living well.

Martyn Evans
Pekka Louhiala
Raimo Puustinen
January 2004

About the editors

Martyn Evans is Professor of Humanities in Medicine at the University of Durham, and Principal of John Snow College at the University. He is joint editor of the *Medical Humanities* editions of the *Journal of Medical Ethics*. He has published variously on the aesthetics of music, ethics and philosophy of medicine, and the role of humanities in medical education. His current interests concern the role of humanities in medical education. When not being a philosopher he is a musician and, when time allows, a dinghy sailor. He is married with two sons; his wife Janet is a professional pianist.

Pekka Louhiala is a lecturer in medical ethics at the University of Helsinki, Finland. He has degrees both in medicine and philosophy and he also works as a part-time paediatrician in private practice. He has published on various topics in medical ethics, philosophy of medicine and epidemiology. His current academic interests include conceptual and philosophical aspects of issues like evidence-based medicine, alternative medicine and placebo.

Raimo Puustinen is a full-time private general practitioner in Tampere, central Finland, and a part-time lecturer at the University of Tampere Medical School. He is a member of the editorial board of *Medical Humanities*. His publications cover the anthropology, ethics and philosophy of medicine and the role of humanities in medical theory, and he has also co-authored an introductory book on general practice for medical students and a book on the essence of medicine for a lay audience. His media work includes almost 300 appearances on a health programme on Finnish national TV, and various radio appearances on health matters. His current interests concern problems in medical theory from a semiotic viewpoint. His musical interests include playing tenor sax and blues harp. He is married with four children; his wife Aino is a professional weaver.

List of contributors

Pentti Alanen
Professor of Community Dentistry
Institute of Dentistry
University of Turku
Finland

Shinik Kang
Researcher
Department of Medical History and Ethics
Ilsanpaik Hospital School of Medicine
South Korea

John Saunders
Consultant Physician and Honorary Research Fellow
Centre for Philosophy and Health Care (University of Wales Swansea)
Nevill Hall Hospital
Wales

William Stempsey
Associate Professor of Philosophy
College of the Holy Cross
Worcester, Massachusetts
United States

Pekka Vuoria
Professor Emeritus
University of Oulu
Finland

Heikki S Vuorinen
Researcher
Department of Public Health
Finland

Paul Wainwright
Reader in Humanities and Health Care
Centre for Philosophy, Humanities and Law in Health Care
University of Wales Swansea
Wales

Acknowledgements

The seminar from which this book grew was held at the University of Wales Gregynog, Powys, Wales, in the Spring of 2001. It was made possible only by the support of the University of Wales Gregynog, The University of Wales Research Colloquium Fund, and The Nuffield Trust – we owe our thanks to all of these. We gratefully acknowledge also the support provided by the University of Helsinki, the University of Joensuu, and the University of Tampere, who together enabled the participation of a number of colleagues from Finland. The original idea for a book of this kind was conceived by Professors Pekka Vuoria and William Stempsey, and we are indebted to them both for this and for their contributions to this volume – as we are, of course, to all our contributing authors, a number of whom were also participants at the Gregynog seminar. Finally, we acknowledge the debts each of us has to our students, past and present.

The day begins ...

'Oh, no ... Doctor, I'm really sorry ...'

'OK, OK, my fault, I should have been looking out – how about a swab?'

'No, you're really bleeding there, Doctor – er, that looks nasty.'

'Yeah, hey, that is bleeding ... OK, I'd better quit. Quick – call Dr Donoghue and ask if she can find someone to take over from here. Put a clamp on there, and there ...'

The doctor, a surgical registrar, walked to the dressing room and pulled off his blood-sodden left surgical glove. The cut gaped, and blood flowed freely. He held his hand under the cold tap for several minutes as the flesh slowly went numb.

As the pain subsided he began to feel slightly nauseous. He was glad when a senior colleague came into the dressing room, and installed himself at the adjoining basin to scrub up.

'Ouch, looks nasty. How did you manage that?'

'Oh, I don't know, nothing really – I just got a cut from a scalpel as it was being passed to me. My fault – I was looking the wrong way.'

'Some cut! You need that stitched. Get along to Casualty – now. And this happened during surgery? The patient was already opened up? Any blood contact?'

'Er, yeah, suppose so.'

'OK, let's be smart. Follow procedure. Check the records. Is the patient clean? Then get your blood checked at the lab. Here, let's have a proper look at that cut ... that is nasty. Look, you know you're not going to be operating for a while? Got that? Tell them to cancel your list for a couple of weeks at least. On second thoughts, I'll tell them.'

As his colleague left, the registrar rolled some dressing around his hand, changed out of his surgical gown and headed off to Casualty, with sensation returning rapidly and painfully to his left thumb.

The pain got worse while he was waiting for the lift. His thumb became stiff and swollen. He remembered that he had promised to go fishing with his son over the weekend. And new kitchen cupboard doors were waiting to be installed.

'What a mess, and with just one thumb,' he thought as he got into the lift.

First let's consider your left thumb ...
An introduction to the philosophy of medicine

Martyn Evans

A strange invitation

Please take a long, hard look at your left thumb. For most people, that is easy enough – just look, and there it is.[1] Well, I'm assuming that with this left thumb of yours you are probably now gripping this book and its pages, so in the ordinary run of things it is an important practical help to you in reading this chapter.

That grip and your left thumb's role in it are things that you normally take for granted when reading. Even so, please take just a few moments to look at your thumb, sense it and feel it. Focus your consciousness momentarily on – or 'in' – your left thumb. Take your thumb seriously! And when you have done that and are ready to read on, see if you can retain some sense of your left thumb's presence and importance when you are reading.

This whole book is about philosophy – in quite a broad sense, although very definitely applied to medicine. There are many definitions of philosophy, but for my purposes in this chapter I would like to suggest that philosophy is actually about *not* taking for granted at least one of the things that we normally take for granted about reading. If you can

---

[1] At least, I hope that 'there it is'. Perhaps not every reader of this book has a left thumb, so a special apology for this example is owed to anyone who lacks a left thumb. I hope that the enquiries contained in this chapter will still be of interest to such readers.

manage it, I would like you *not* to take for granted – on just this one occasion – your left thumb's role in your reading.

About a left thumb – but not yours

Before we start to think about your left thumb, I'm going to tell you a few things about my own. A few of these things will apply to your thumb as well, but most will not. To begin with, my thumb is more or less the size and shape you would expect from looking at the rest of my left hand. As for its general colour, you would tell that from looking at me as a whole. I have the general colour of a caucasian skin, which for some reason we call 'white', but it is obviously nothing at all like white. As well as this general colour, like most thumbs it sees more of the sun than, say, my left big toe, so it has a slight tan on the back (i.e. the nail side). The nail itself is ridged and, like all of my fingernails, slightly 'clubbed' or convex. My doctor has been interested in this 'clubbing' in the past, but fortunately for me it turned out not to matter in the way he at first thought.

The creases in the skinfolds over the knuckle joint are quite thick. When I was a teenager I had eczema on my hands, and the skin has coarsened a little, making my hands look perhaps slightly older than my 47 years. A number of marks and small scratches on my thumb would tell a detective or a pathologist that I do some practical tasks, including minor repairs to my motorbike, a small amount of woodworking, odd jobs in the garden, and so on. A forensic specialist would be able to tell even more about the type of woodworking I do. There is a faint purplish tan on part of the 'ball' of the thumbtip, where the acid in my sweat has etched the steel in a special tool called a cabinet-scraper, which I use when working with hard woods such as oak or ash. However, my hands do not have the permanently shiny, grimy appearance of someone who does these things all day every day, professionally. My thumb is still the thumb of someone who spends most of his day at a desk, but who 'relaxes' with a spanner or a saw in his hands.

Near the base of my thumb is a small half-moon-shaped white scar. When I was four years old I tripped over a toy while I was carrying a glass dish. The dish broke and the glass cut me deeply. I have no mental picture of the accident itself, but I clearly remember the medical consultation at the physician's surgery and the frequent changing of complicated gauze dressings for many days afterwards. The memory of the raw interior faces of the cut slices of flesh, moving against each other with a sickening tenderness no matter how gently the doctor (or the nurse, or later even my mother) lifted off the old, matted, blood-encrusted gauze, comes to my mind right now. Or rather, it comes to my mind, my stomach and my thumb itself, for the memory of that dreadful tugging sensation 'lives' even now in my left thumb – the thumb is itself the bearer of a kind of memory.

When I look at my left thumb at this moment, resting on the keyboard of my computer, I see that it is trembling slightly. It tells me that I am tired after arriving home late last night from a meeting in London, that I have been typing rapidly with many repetitive movements, that I have been drinking strong coffee, and that I have a rather poor ability to relax my muscles generally. It even tells me that I am beginning to feel a little of that anticipation and excitement that comes with settling down to start writing something which I have been putting off for too long, and which might perhaps be worth writing. However, the trembling also reminds me that despite my occupation as a professional philosopher, I am more authentically *myself* (if such a strange phrase makes any sense) when I am acting physically, purposefully and above all fluently than when I am resting and contemplating. There is, of course, action, as well as fluency of a kind, involved in typing at the computer. However, this action is constantly interrupted by thinking and working out what it is I actually want to say. By contrast, my thumb becomes most fully and fluently *itself* when I play the piano. By 'itself', I mean my thumb in the state when it feels most natural to me, and when my conscious awareness of it – and of the world *through* it – is at its most acute and meaningful. My left thumb, as it happens, is more prominent in my piano playing than my right thumb, because it can be used to project the melodies that sometimes appear in what we could call the 'middle' of the sound space used on the piano keyboard – the notes that would be sung by the tenors in a choir. The composer Johannes Brahms actually used to speak of his own left thumb as his 'tenor thumb', and he considered it to be one of his most important resources in his own piano playing and composing. Well, to me it feels that projecting these tenor notes through a rich, satisfying, highly physical engagement with the keys is the time when my own left thumb's nature is best fulfilled – if you like, what my left thumb is *for*.

This chapter is supposed to be about *your* left thumb, and not about mine, so I will not continue the autobiography much longer. There is more that I could say – or, rather, there is more that my left thumb could say about me. However, it might be worth mentioning right now that if the accident with the glass dish had left my thumb paralysed, or severed, or so badly damaged that it was useless or required amputation, then some of the things which I now do and which are so important to me as to be actually *constitutive* of me (especially playing the piano, perhaps) would not have been possible in the way that they are. I happen to be left-handed. Presumably I would have had to learn to write with my right hand, but I doubt whether I could have learned to draw or paint with my right hand. Probably there are motorcyclists who have no left thumb, but I cannot imagine riding safely if I lost the use of mine now. I would, of course, have been able to take up different interests, but in choosing them I would not have taken my thumbs for granted. And in doing different things I would have become, I think, a slightly different 'me'. In his novel *The English Patient*, Michael Ondaatje shows us a man who is changed by the loss of his thumbs. 'Caravaggio', the intelligence agent whose thumbs are cut off by the Nazis, becomes a kind of fugitive from his own perception of himself, addicted to morphine in the headlong flight from his physical and 'existential' pain.

I said earlier that philosophy is about *not* taking for granted the things that we usually *do* take for granted. Evidently I myself have not been very philosophical about my thumb until the time came to think about writing this chapter. Before I began to write it, I can see now that I too had taken my left thumb completely and utterly for granted. Moreover, I have tended to take for granted the things that I do. It can sometimes seem to us that we freely choose the things that we do, as if we wandered into a supermarket of activities and interests, hobbies and occupations, and chose things from the shelves. However, life is not like that, as a moment's (philosophical) reflection will tell us. Some choices are open to us and others are not open to us, and these reflect our physical endowment. For example, I was never big, strong or skilful enough to play soccer for my school team. And then they come to be reflected *in* us. For example, my very identity, by now, is in a strong sense bound up with the things that I habitually do (writing, playing the piano, making things from wood, steering a little wooden sailing-boat) and which, as it happens, require my left thumb to function in the way that it does.

My left thumb is thus 'part of me' in more than one sense. It is physically part of me, but it is also personally, biographically, part of me – part of the story about me and part of the ingredients which make the story possible, which determine what sort of story there *could* be about me.

And, if you have one, the same is true about your left thumb.

And now about your own left thumb

So far we have been thinking about things that are true in particular about a particular thumb. You can tell a story of exactly this kind about your own left thumb. Obviously I cannot tell that particular story. However, there remains a more general story which together we can tell, as philosophers, about your thumb. This story is to do with some very general facts about our common experience as embodied humans – facts that are, in my opinion, philosophically vital to clinical medicine.

So the rest of this chapter will concern these facts, this more general story and this common experience. In telling it, it is more important to think about your left thumb than to think about mine. In thinking about it, let us try not to take for granted the things that we normally might take for granted.

Looking and touching

To begin with, if you are reading this chapter unaided, and if you have a left thumb, and if it is not temporarily hidden by a glove or a bandage, then obviously you can see your thumb. But is your thumb the very same thumb that I could see if we were sitting in the same room together and I looked at it? In an important sense, the answer must be 'no'. For me, your thumb is one of the many objects in the world about me. And for you, the same would be true of *my* thumb. However, your own thumb is not like this, *for you*. Your thumb is not simply one more object among the many objects that you can see in the world around you. Capturing this in words is not easy – we fall back in to saying things such as your thumb is attached to you, it is part of you, it *is* you. These things are true, but we do not always appreciate either their depth or, as I shall try to show, their mystery.

When you look at your thumb, in an important sense you look at yourself. Your thumb is capable of telling the kind of individual story about you which my thumb told about myself, a few lines ago. However, the 'telling' has, for you, an intimacy and an immediacy which it cannot have for other people. When you look at your thumb, you look at part of the way in which you are physically extended into the world. If some aspects of your immediate surroundings are physically hostile (cold, hot, on fire, electrically charged, highly acid, sharp-edged, abrasive and so on), then your thumb is for you a plainly vulnerable extension of your experience. It is a living part of that surface network of your nerve endings which in the wrong circumstances can confront you directly and immediately with discomfort or pain. In extreme circumstances that network can turn your world into a living hell, and your left thumb is a continuous part of that world-changing possibility. You are, of course, careful where you put your thumb. However, a fuller way of saying this is to say that you are careful where you put your*self*, including that part of your self which is your thumb.

Thus, consciously or otherwise, when you look at your thumb all of this vulnerability, caution and sensitivity is a part of what you know, and therefore a part of what you *see*. You know that this is true of other people's thumbs, for them – but you know that theoretically, abstractly.

For your own thumb you know it immediately. Your thumb is not another object merely within the world – it is part of what your world is.

We can say pretty much the same about your other sensory perception of your thumb – your perception 'of' your thumb in the sense of 'directed towards' it, as for example when you look at it. Most importantly, consider your ability to touch your left thumb with your other fingers or your other hand. With them you can touch, sense and feel your left thumb, but of course normally you also at the same time feel *with* it, or through it – you sense the touching in the thumb itself, as well as in the part that touches it. You might sometimes put your hand against a child's forehead to tell whether or not he or she has a raised temperature. However, that same hand placed against your own forehead is somehow no longer able to give you such information. Your forehead tells you the temperature of your hand at the same time as your hand tells you of the temperature of your forehead, and somehow the resultant information is garbled, or fused together.

Again, the 'taken-for-grantedness' of this is startling, and we notice it only when the normal circumstances of touch are altered. Specifically, to touch a part of yourself that has been numbed with local anaesthetic is an eerie and to some extent horrible experience. For an important part of what makes your thumb part of yourself is the 'feedback' that it gives you through touch. If your thumb is locally anaesthetised, touching it is – revoltingly – like touching an alien thumb, something that ought to be part of you but which is not, at least for the moment. Suddenly the thumb seems to be reduced to being just another of the many objects in the world around you, and they are definitely not part of you. Provided they are not dangerous, out of reach or socially forbidden, you can touch most of the things in the world around you. (that world includes other people, of course, and interpersonal touching is a crucial but delicate aspect of clinical medicine). However, your thumb in its ordinary, non-anaesthetised state is not one of the things in the world around you. It is indeed in the world, but whereas the book you are now holding is in the world in precisely the same sense for you as it is for me – it is a common object in both of our worlds – your thumb is not. Your thumb, like your body as a whole, is part of the *medium* of your world – it is part of how the world is presented to you.

Doing and acting

Your thumb, like your body as a whole, is also part of how you present yourself to the world, and part of how you do things in the world – how you act, undertake and accomplish. Soon you will turn the next page of this book. Using your left thumb, you carefully press a little bulge in the edge of the stack of unread pages on the right-hand side of the open book, probably pinching the open face of that page with your left index finger, and you slip your thumb in behind the bulge and peel off the next page towards the already read pages on the left.

If your hands are unimpaired, you did this with unconscious fluency – accurately, effectively. You will have had uncounted hours of practice at this since childhood. Children find this task quite difficult at first – as if they are trying to follow instructions based on the type of rather tortuous description I have just given. Physically it is probably quite a skilled task – probably more skilled than putting an outer cover on a duvet (something that many adults find absorbingly difficult to do, and for which a university education somehow never quite seems to prepare us).

What was your thumb's 'job' in this fairly complicated page-turning manoeuvre? Here I do not mean to ask about the physical description as such, but rather I mean to ask about the relationship between your intention to turn the page and the actions that your thumb actually performed. You are now reading the second (third, etc.) page of this chapter. So you have successfully turned the page, and you did it skilfully – and *wilfully* (that is, intentionally). What happened (the turning of the page) did so because you wanted it to. It was an act of will. Yet the act itself was so automatic and inevitable that you probably gave it no conscious thought, and the 'thinking' took place, as it were, in your muscles and tendons, on the skin surface and in the nerve endings of your thumb- and fingertips. It would become difficult to do it fluently if you *were* thinking about it, just as walking becomes next to impossible if you give yourself 'instructions' on the sequence of bodily movements involved and try to carry them out. However, even if it is done 'automatically' or unconsciously in this sense, if the action is performed in order to achieve a result then it is natural to say that it was intended.

Consciously thinking about our body parts often leads to a strange kind of immobility in them, a sort of temporary functional interruption. It might be interesting to see whether you are able to turn the next page in quite the same unconsciously fluent way now that I have drawn your attention to it. Interestingly, there is a type of symmetry about this, in that if your left thumb becomes impaired for some other reason (for example, because it is stiff, sore, broken, enervated or anaesthetised, or is actually missing), then at least to begin with you really do have to think about your movements in a way that would ordinarily be quite disabling. You have to recalculate and relearn your actions before they can become fluent and unconscious.

There is both a medical/therapeutic question and a philosophical question here. The medical question is to do with how we build a bridge between what an ordinary person can ordinarily do, and what a damaged or disabled person has to relearn to do. The philosophical question, which I think is deeply relevant to the medical question, is concerned with how we should ordinarily describe and analyse our actions, so that we have some basis for describing and analysing the predicament facing someone who is damaged or disabled, or – better still – for understanding those descriptions and analyses which the disabled themselves may be in a much better position to provide for us.

Part of the philosophical question concerns something very important about the way in which we experience our actions, whether we are disabled or not. Do we act freely and intentionally? And are our actions the expressions of our free will? These slightly crazy-sounding questions are important for medicine well beyond the management of disability. Most obviously, the whole business of rational diagnosis and judgement in medicine relies on the idea that we can work things out for ourselves, and then go and act on the basis of the answers that we come up with. And the whole of our experience of our embodied existence is that within certain limits we *are* free, and we *do* make intentional choices and act upon them. Now if the answers to the crazy-sounding questions are a simple 'yes' – and common sense and daily experience seem to require that they be exactly that – why bother raising the questions at all? Well, your left thumb might show us why.

When you turned the page, was your thumb putting your intention into effect? Initially you are probably tempted to say 'yes'. So was it a sort of tool or instrument for you – an instrument of your will? Still you might be tempted to answer, 'yes', although this expression 'instrument of your will' is not a very natural-sounding one. However, the obvious alternatives (it has a will of its own, it is the instrument of someone else's will, or it acts haphazardly and uncontrolledly) seem even less natural. The trouble is that, on analysis, none of the ordinary ways of speaking about this seem to be as clearly understood as we might like them to be.

From the scientific point of view we could ask 'What caused the page to move?'. Among other things, your thumb did. But what caused your thumb to move? Muscles and tendons, of course. But what caused *them* to move? Nerve impulses, you reply. But what caused *them* to move? Now we seem uncertain about how to respond. Outside the world of the physical and life sciences we know how to respond. We stop talking about causes. We say, 'Never mind about the nerve impulses. My thumb moved because I moved it. And I moved it because I meant to. I moved it intentionally – that's why it moved.' However, from the viewpoint of medical science this looks rather evasive. Indeed, the difficulty lies in saying *from the scientific point of view* exactly what and where your intention is to be found, other than somehow in the action itself. Even you yourself could not find the intention anywhere else – you could not see it or feel it. Yet almost inescapably you believe in it – in general, we believe that we do things because we mean to do them. Even as I type these words, I find that I am wholly convinced by the belief that I shall type exactly the letters I choose, so long as I am careful! And what more intentional, deliberate behaviour could there be than 'taking care'? Thus it seems to follow from this that it is my *intention* that is finally responsible for the physical movements of my fingers and thumbs, even if I am not actively supervising the traffic along my neural and muscular pathways. And of course I am not doing *that*. The trouble is that 'intention' is not something that science can easily describe, or even observe.

Science deals comfortably with mechanisms, and I admit that there is an undeniably mechanical *aspect* to our structure and function. So is your thumb's movement the movement of a mechanism? At the skeletal and muscular level, perhaps it seems like that. However, the problem of what *causes* the movement in the first place remains. You move your thumb by an act of will, albeit one that cost you no thought or effort. Yet an 'act of will' is, it seems, the description of something mental. So how does a mental event produce or cause a physical result? The page obtains its movement – kinetic energy – from the thumb. But from where does the thumb gain *its* energy? To talk in terms of actin and myosin and sugars and oxygen only pushes back the problem. What actuated them? What made it possible for them to be actuated precisely now for just exactly the intended result? There seems to be no alternative to saying that it was the intention itself – an essential mental phenomenon. So now, finally, what (or where) is the interaction between the mental and the physical? There must be *some* link, we want to say – otherwise we could not move beyond an intention to the point of actually producing an action. And our experience seems to confirm that we can intend to perform an action and achieve it. When we are healthy, it almost seems as if we can do this whenever we want – within the range of what we think is normally possible for us.

Well, let us indulge what we want to say – 'But there must be *some* link'. Have we 'explained' how your left thumb moved? In one sense, we have not. If, in the language of physical science, we say that your thumb's movement was caused *simply* within the material or mechanical world, with nothing left over, then we seem to have lost your intention, your purpose. If it was nothing more than a physical event, your thumb's movement could be a mechanical affair which we could have predicted on physical grounds alone, the same being true, inevitably, for all of our bodily actions. In this case, our will is either detached from the mechanism, playing no genuine role in it, or must itself be part of the mechanism – a further part of the material world.

If it is detached from the mechanical world and plays no role in it, then 'free will' is just a delusion. It happens to *feel* to us as if free will were real, but we are just kidding ourselves. However, everything in us protests against this. We cannot – at least when we are healthy – seriously accept that our desire to keep reading has no other connection with our thumb's turning of the page than some kind of happy and regular coincidence. We seem forced, paradoxically, to think of ourselves as free! At any rate we have no everyday alternative to experiencing 'free will' as real.

If, on the other hand, free will is itself a 'part of the physical mechanism', then why have the neurologists not found it and isolated and described it? Since it has certainly resisted scientific observation and explanation so far, is it just more complicated or harder to see under a microscope? Or is it the wrong kind of thing altogether to be pursuing with a microscope (as though searching for it under a microscope would be a mistake, like searching for *the taste* of chocolate in a brain scan of someone who was eating a chocolate bar)?

Our experience of free will is so vividly real that it seems complete nonsense to regard the term 'free will' as merely the name of some widespread delusion. Indeed, to speak of delusion at all is to talk about something that we experience, in life lived 'from the inside', and something we can ordinarily tell apart from reality – ideas which make no sense if the mind is not real, or if free will is not a reality. So your left thumb and its role in turning that page have drawn our attention to a problem which is very important when we remember that medicine is above all a science of the human. Intentions seem to us, in our ordinary everyday experience, to be central to our actions as humans. Yet if medicine confines itself to a basis in science, it will not be able to recognise, still less understand, this central feature of action. However, disturbances or obstacles to action are a major reason why people go to see their doctors.

Analysing and repairing

In order to repair something, we need to have at least some understanding of how it works and what it is made of. If your thumb hurts, or is weak, broken, paralysed or disfigured, then your normal response is to seek help from medicine. And medicine asks the following question. What is your thumb, *biologically speaking?* Here anatomy, physiology and neurology combine to give a wonderfully detailed account of its structure, properties and compositional fabric. However, sooner or later we have to face a truth which we often overlook, probably because it is uncomfortable. Eventually we have to admit that your thumb is *meat*, yet it is a piece of that extraordinary kind of meat of which we ourselves are ultimately composed.

The extraordinary thing about us is, of course, that we are meat which feels, thinks, and knows that it feels and thinks; meat that experiences the world from the inside. In short, to use a phrase that I find helpful, we are 'meat with a point of view'! This uncomfortable recognition invites a further (and I think important philosophical) question, namely what it is we want from medicine – what it is we want out doctors to do. When you consult a doctor to deal with the problem in your thumb, do you seek a change in the meat's nature? Or do you seek a change in your experience of it? Or do you seek a change in your viewpoint of the world and your thumb's place in it? Do you seek a change in the physical world or in your experience of it, or in both?

This is partly a matter of what you think the doctor is competent to try to change, or to repair. If your thumb is stiff, painful, broken, paralysed or missing altogether, the doctor's response may be to a thumb that is impaired, or to a function that is impaired, or to a person who is impaired. The focus of doctors' training in the scientific era inclines them heavily towards looking first of all at the substance of the thumb itself. When they look at its function, their training inclines them to look at function more in terms of normal and abnormal physiology, and much less in terms of the patient's experience of the world and the place in that experience of the body as a whole, including the thumb and all of its perceptual and 'historical' contributions (as I have outlined them in this chapter) to the patient's experience and the patient's world.

If 'health' means that the parts of your body meet the expectations of statistical norms, then a mechanical approach to diagnosis and treatment is perfectly appropriate. However, if 'health' means something more like your ability to experience and engage with the world in a way that you are used to, understand and enjoy, then this has the most profound implications for the preparation, training and post-qualification education of clinical doctors. From our point of view in this chapter (and indeed in this book as a whole), our recognition that clinical medicine is bristling with philosophical questions suggests that doctors gain much, and perhaps offer much to their patients subsequently, when they recognise and reflect on these questions in a philosophical spirit. I am sure that there have always been doctors who have done this – not least because these questions have always been at the heart of clinical medicine, and have always called forth the spirit of philosophical enquiry. Because it is perhaps harder to make time for such enquiry in the highly technicised form of medicine that we have in our own day, it seems more important than ever to encourage our doctors to retain their philosophical curiosity.

Wondering and being amazed

As a philosopher, my own reflections lead me to a sense of wonderment at the mystery of our embodied nature. I wish that there was more time for that sense of wonder in the average doctor's daily professional practice, intervening in the perspective and the fabric of these living, breathing, walking pieces of meat, each with their own point of view. However, whether or not there is time for it, that sense of wonder seems to me inevitably to have a *stake* in daily clinical practice. And the broadly philosophical questions that we have encountered, recognised and considered are, in my view, always prompted by the clinical consultation – whether silently or aloud, spurned or acknowledged. Whether or not we have answers to these questions, it is curious to note how they have been prompted by nothing more – and, fantastically, wonderfully, nothing *less* – than that remarkable and mysterious piece of human fabric which is your left thumb.

'Right, let's have a look.'

The duty doctor peeled off the dressing and scrutinised the injured thumb.

'Mmmm, it's nasty. How on earth did you manage that?'

'Just lost concentration.'

The duty doctor reached for a syringe. The registrar bit his lip as his thumb was being anaesthetised.

'OK, a few stitches and it'll be fine. Can you move the thumb at all? How far? Yeah, well the tendons seem to be intact. You'll be operating again in a week.'

The duty doctor cut the thread and called a nurse to put on a dressing, which turned the thumb into a smart white truncheon of bandage. The nurse went away, leaving the registrar feeling very tired and alone.

'Now what?', he wondered.

And then the doctor told me ...
The clinical encounter as the core of medicine

Raimo Puustinen

Introduction

Doctors are often criticised for not listening to their patients. It has been claimed that doctors do not have adequate communication skills and that they should attend communication courses to enable them to respond better to their patients' problems. This might be true in the sense that perhaps we would all benefit from having better communication skills. However, it seems that there is more involved than just skills and courtesy in the question of how doctors communicate with their patients.

I am more than willing to believe that doctors do, in general, listen to their patients carefully. However, the question is 'What do they attend to when they listen to their patients' complaints?'. And this raises the question of how we should understand the doctor's task, since it is what they attend to that ultimately guides the way in which doctors approach their patients' problems and complaints.

The structure and conduct of a medical consultation may, at the outset, seem fairly simple. A patient approaches a doctor and complains of the symptoms of feeling ill. After a brief conversation, the doctor performs a physical examination. The doctor then infers the nature of the patient's problem from the information gathered, establishes a diagnosis and prescribes a treatment. However, straightforward as it may seem, this brief encounter consists of a vast number of theoretical and practical problems – from the patient's first experience of malaise, to the decision to seek medical advice, to the medical diagnosis and treatment, and finally to eventual recovery, chronic illness or death.

The medical consultation has attracted increasing academic interest, especially among social scientists and linguists (Pendleton, 1986; Korsch *et al.*, 1995). Despite the many elegant studies which have been performed, there is still no agreed theoretical framework bringing all of the various aspects of the phenomenon into focus. However, there have been attempts to develop a theory of medicine based on the medical consultation as the essence of medicine. In what follows, I shall examine some basic features of these approaches and discuss their implications for the philosophy of medicine.

The craft of signs

Ancient doctors called their craft a *techne semeiotike*, referring to the skill of interpreting signs (Baer, 1988). This definition incorporates three aspects of the medical consultation. First, it points to the problem of deciphering signs and symptoms in medicine. Secondly, the term *techne* refers to the conduct of medical practice. Thirdly, the medical consultation is by definition an interpersonal phenomenon – it is a communicative act between two human individuals, namely the doctor and the patient.

In the Hippocratic writings, the problem of interpreting a patient's signs and symptoms were addressed as follows:

> [The] doctor must have recourse to reasoning from the symptoms with which he is presented .... The symptoms which patients describe to their doctor are based on guesses about a possible cause rather than knowledge about it.
>
> (Lloyd, 1983, pp. 145–7)

A doctor's task was thus understood to be the structuring of the patient's vague observations and interpretations about his or her ill-being within a theory of disease that the doctor followed in his or her practice. To achieve this, the doctor must observe the signs of disease. However, these signs are not always readily perceptible, and may sometimes need to be produced by an active intervention.

> When the doctor cannot make an exact diagnosis from the patient's description of his symptoms, the doctor must employ other methods for his guidance. By weighing up the significance of various [bodily] signs, it is possible to deduce of what disease they are the result .... .

Even when nature herself does not produce such signs, they may be revealed by certain harmless measures known to those practised in the science.

(1983, pp. 145–7)

The practical difficulties which follow from the overwhelming number and variability of potential signs in each and every case are also well recognised by the ancient writers:

But both the methods to be employed and the signs produced differ from case to case. As a result, the signs may be difficult for the doctor to interpret ... the practitioners of medicine differ greatly among themselves both in theory and practice, just as happens in every other science.

(Lloyd, 1983, p. 70)

These fundamental problems of medical practice have not vanished with the development of modern medicine (or biomedicine, as it is commonly called). Although contemporary medicine is held to be a branch of natural science, dominated by an empiricist viewpoint (Wulff *et al.*, 1990), the problem of eliciting and interpreting the patient's signs and symptoms during a medical consultation is as central to a scientifically trained doctor as it was to his or her ancient predecessors.

Contemporary medical research generally addresses clinical phenomena using quantitative terms and methods. This derives from the idea that the human body is a biological phenomenon, where different functions and structures can be measured and expressed in such physical and chemical concepts as millimetres of mercury, millimoles per litre or cubic centimetres. However, during a medical consultation the doctor is repeatedly confronted by a variety of human phenomena that cannot be approached or solved by the methods of biological sciences alone. Many of these phenomena therefore need to be expressed and dealt with in qualitative terms – (for instance, 'unemployed', 'depression', 'alcoholism', 'jaundice', etc.) (Evans, 1998). Qualitative methods and the humanities are therefore increasingly employed in medical research and education (Simpson *et al.*, 1991; Green and Britten, 1998). The growing interest in the conduct of the medical consultation can be seen as part of a broader tendency to enlarge our view of the nature and goals of medicine in general, and to develop the theory of medicine to correspond more closely with clinical phenomena as they are encountered in everyday medical practice.

The 'Bio-psycho-social' model of medicine

In 1978, Georg Engel, an American internist and psychiatrist, published his still influential paper on 'The need for a new medical model: a challenge for biomedicine' (Engel, 1978). In his essay, Engel discussed how the current biomedical model of medicine embraces both *reductionism* (the philosophical view that complex phenomena are ultimately derived from a single primary principle) and *mind–body dualism* (the doctrine that fundamentally separates the mind from the body). The reductionist principle in biomedical thinking is *physicalist* by nature – that is, it assumes that the language of the physical sciences (chemistry and physics) will suffice to explain biological and ultimately medical phenomena.

According to Engel, a more comprehensive understanding of a disease as a human phenomenon requires additional concepts and frames of reference. For instance, the way in which diabetic symptoms are experienced and the way in which they are reported by any one individual all require consideration of psychological, social, cultural and other concurrent complicating factors.

Establishing a relationship between the specific biochemical processes of a particular patient's illness requires a scientifically rational approach to the behavioural and psychosocial data, for these are the terms in which most clinical phenomena are reported by patients. In addition, with the application of rational therapies it needs to be acknowledged how powerfully the behaviour of the doctor, as well as the relationship between patient and doctor, influence the therapeutic outcome for better or for worse.

Engel has proposed a *bio-psycho-social model* of medicine to bring together the various aspects of medical theory and practice. The model is based on general *systems theory*, in which reality is considered to be built on hierarchical levels which differ in their degree of complexity, and where the upper level presupposes the lower one. Engel's model retains the *biological* basis of medicine, but it suggests that we need to increase the number of variables which should be taken into account in medical practice. These variables are derived from different scientific disciplines' concepts and methods of addressing the world. Thus according to the bio-psycho-social model, medicine is seen as a mixture of scientific disciplines applied by a doctor to the care of the patient.

In his later writings, Engel examined the features of the medical consultation more closely. According to Engel, within the clinical consultation the doctor acts as a *participant observer* who, in the process of attending to the patient's complaints, taps into his or her own personal inner viewing system in order to compare and clarify the data obtained from the patient.

However, the patient is both an initiator and a collaborator in the process, not merely an object of study. The three basic components of the method for clinical study consist of *observation* (outer viewing) *introspection* (inner viewing), and *dialogue* (interviewing), and these components eventually convert the data from the patient into a scientific form (Engel, 1997).

The medical consultation establishes the conditions and framework within which scientific work with patients proceeds. Thus the clinical encounter is not an obstacle to objectivity on the part of the doctor, but rather it is another mode of data collection. In the clinical setting, the scientific effort becomes a joint undertaking to be negotiated between the doctor and the patient. The doctor as a scientist operates concurrently in two modes, namely an observational mode in which the patient is approached as an object of the study, and a relational mode in which the relationship between the patient and the doctor actually modifies the data obtained.

Engel assumes that once we acknowledge how fundamental the dialogue is within the consultation, the essential complementarity of the human and the scientific will become apparent. This is part and parcel of the fact that dialogue as a means of data collection and processing is *itself* regulated by the conditions which determine human relationships in general (Engel, 1992).

The key to the psychosocial realm within the medical encounter lies in the nature of human relationships, whose essential medium is *dialogue*. According to Engel, the clinical interview is the most powerful, comprehensive, sensitive and versatile instrument available to the doctor. It is the 'scientific instrument' for investigating the human realm in medicine (Engel, 1997).

For Engel, the search for a scientific model for medicine ultimately rests on the issue of whether, in studying and caring for their patients, doctors can *also* be scientists and work scientifically in the human domain. Thus it seems that, for Engel, the fundamental distinction is not the simple one between 'science' and 'art', but rather that between those who think and proceed scientifically in medicine and those who do not.

The idea of 'the person' as medicine's object

Another attempt to develop medical theory so as to correspond more closely to everyday medical practice is Eric Cassel's introduction of the concept of 'the person' as medicine's object of inquiry. For Cassel, medicine is about the care of the sick, and all medical care flows through the relationship between doctor and patient (Cassel, 1984). The core of medicine is the consultation, in which the doctor should approach the patient as a person, rather than as a mere biological phenomenon. As Cassel himself has formulated it:

> the focus of medicine is the sick person … the individual sick person is both our concern and under our direct observation.
>
> (Cassel, 1991, p. 155)

When the *person* is established as the logically central point of concern in medicine, then scientific information about disease and technology becomes subservient to that person's own interests. Thus clinical theory needs to place the person (sick or well) at the centre of the doctor's thoughts, without impairing the doctor's ability to think or act scientifically (Cassel, 1997).

According to Cassel, it is nothing more than dogma in modern medicine to suppose that knowing what to do with the sick consists merely of understanding the biological mechanism involved in the illness. In clinical medical *practice*, there is a genuine need also to understand the doctor's actions, the relationship between doctor and patient, and other non-scientific areas of medicine (Cassel, 1984).

Cassel proposes that the person (sick or well) must displace disease as the conceptual and logical centre of the system of medicine. Thinking about medicine should always focus one's mind upon the patient. The patient is at medicine's conceptual core, reaching upward to the community and downward to his or her molecules. Everything is logically connected to the patient, who in a sense represents human beings in general, and stands for each and every dimension of being human – including the dimensions of being healthy, sick *or* 'diseased'.

For Cassel, spoken language is the most important tool in medicine, and almost no diagnostic or therapeutic act takes place without it. During a consultation, the patient tells his or her history while the doctor elicits, records and interprets this particular history. The clinician is not gathering isolated facts each of which is separate from the others or from the whole. Rather, the pertinent facts are tied together by the meanings with which they are imbued – meanings that are specific to the patient, the doctor, and the culture that they both share. It is ultimately, the *meanings* of objects, relationships and events – not isolated and singular facts – that drive the actions of the patient and the doctor.

Medicine as a human practice

Our third example of an attempt to place medical consultation at the heart of medical theory is Edmund Pellegrino's philosophy of medicine, in which medicine is seen as a form of human interaction between doctor and patient in pursuit of healing.

In their book *A Philosophical Basis of Medical Practice*, Edmund Pellegrino and David Thomasma present the view that medicine is oriented towards caring for human beings. This orientation becomes manifest in medical practice. Thus philosophy of medicine should be developed from the practice of medicine itself, and the practice of medicine should be at the root of all theoretical considerations. For Pellegrino:

> it is in the nature of the healing relationship that we will find what is unique about clinical medicine, what is its immediate end and what will serve as its architectonic principle.
>
> (Pellegrino, 1983, p. 155)

According to Pellegrino and Thomasma (1981), a philosophy of medicine must somehow unite the concreteness of clinical experience with the critical method of philosophy if it is to satisfy both philosophy and medicine. Given the complexity of modern medicine, any philosophy of medicine must be developed from medical practice. The authors choose to be eclectic since, as they argue, no single philosophical stance is capable of a complete exploration of the substance of medicine. However, philosophy of medicine should not be just a philosophical hotchpotch of those sciences and arts that medicine employs. Medicine is not reducible to biology, physics, chemistry or psychology, even in combination, nor is it simply what doctors do or what patients expect, nor is it simply a rigorous science, or alternatively just the art of making good on clinical hunches. Philosophy of medicine is instead a philosophy of an identifiable human activity or practice – a unique form of healing relationship within which a cure may take place.

This theory relies partly on empiricism – that is, an emphasis on the *experiences* of the participants in (and witnesses to) a healing practice. The theory also borrows from phenomenology, such that we focus on the constituent *features* or *phenomena* that medicine characteristically presents to us – the activities, behaviours and relationships that are peculiar to medicine.

Thus the specificity of medicine is located in a human relationship – the relationship of healing in which one person in need of healing seeks out another who professes to heal or to assist in healing. Medical acts tie these two individuals together. It is the nature of these acts in the presence of the healing relationship that gives medicine its special character among human activities.

Since the effectiveness of medicine – with regard to either cure or healing – is embedded in practice, our philosophical method must also begin in practice, and must return to it for its pronouncements to be tested. In other words, a philosophy of medicine must consist of a study and a classification of practice, a search for meaning in the practice of medicine, and specific applications of the results of this search. The goal of the clinical interaction derives straightforwardly from the fact that both the patient and the doctor are intent upon searching either for a cure or for healing – something that is, in most cases, sufficiently immediate as to be obvious.

The medical consultation as the core of medicine

A common feature of the three approaches we have surveyed here, namely those of Engel, Cassell and Pellegrino, is their attempt to rewrite current biologically based medical theory by establishing the medical *consultation* as the core function of medicine. The authors choose to be methodologically eclectic, and they draw their notions mainly from general systems theory, empiricism and phenomenology.

In current biomedical thinking, the object of enquiry in medicine is the human body, seen as a biological phenomenon. The doctor is the enquiring subject, who approaches the patient's body as if it were a biological object. This is obvious in some clinical situations, such as surgical interventions, pathology laboratories and intensive-care units. However, the great majority of medical encounters take place between doctors and patients in ordinary consulting rooms, where both parties are fully conscious and both participate in the diagnostic and therapeutic processes. In these settings, the relationship between the doctor and the patient is not between subject and object but rather between one subject and another. During a consultation, the patient and the doctor jointly focus their attention on the problem that the patient presents as the reason which brought him or her to the surgery. Thus medicine needs to think again about exactly what its 'objects' are, and its relationship to them. Today's doctor can no longer view the suffering patient as an isolated object, but must consider him or her within a far more complex world of suffering (Tauber, 1999).

The goal of the medical consultation is shaped by the concepts that medicine uses to construct its diagnoses. These concepts direct the doctor's understanding of what they are doing with their patients. They spell out the relevant observations to be made and they organise the doctor's reflective thinking, thereby directing their responses to the patient's complaints (Puustinen, 1999a; Leiman and Stiles, 2002). For instance, for a surgeon the true target may be the patient's herniated inter-vertebral disc, while for a psychiatrist the target may be the patient's anxiety and depression when suffering from lower-back pain. Thus the structure of the 'medical alliance' between doctor and patient varies according to the understanding of the problem at hand.

If medicine is seen as a joint activity between the doctor and the patient, what are the implications of this for our understanding of the nature of medicine?

First, the aim of the medical consultation is to explore the sequence of events that has led the patient to consult the doctor in the search for either a cure or alleviation. Examining the patient's body obliges us to recognise that it constantly changes and transforms over time. Thus taking the patient's history means considering the 'natural history' of the body. In that sense, clinical knowledge is essentially *historical* knowledge (Toulmin, 1993).

However, clinical knowledge is also *cultural* knowledge. That is, there needs to be a shared understanding between the doctor and the patient about the *meaning* of the symptoms as they are described, or of the aetiology of the ailment as it emerges. This is an especially sensitive matter in cases where the patient has a different cultural background to that of the doctor (Viljanen, 1999).

Therefore, the doctor's understanding of their patient has a very particular focus – it refers to one particular subject in precisely *his* or *her* particular condition, with all of its attendant features of time and place. This then invites the idea that medicine may belong, in such respects, within the realm of the humanities rather than that of science. Having said this, we must bear in mind that even the distinction between science and the humanities has its own cultural roots. In the Continental scientific tradition, for instance, this distinction is not nearly as clear-cut as it is in the Anglo-Saxon world. The German concept of a science *Wissenschaft* – includes both sciences and humanities, with no clear distinction between the two. Furthermore, the idea that humanities deal essentially with particulars while sciences deal with general laws is not sustainable. The generalised gaze of science does not always apply in modern biology. This is especially the case in such fields as developmental and evolutionary biology, where the historical and contextual character of the phenomena under scientific study is unavoidable (Mayr, 1998). The particularised gaze of the humanities is also incomplete. If a work of literature told us nothing about the world beyond its pages, its interest for us would be very limited.

Analysing the medical consultation as an interpersonal activity requires us to consider both the agent and the 'target' or object of the agent's actions – who is doing what to whom. We have to consider how we 'formulate' the object of our enquiry in medical practice, and how we conceive of, identify and obtain the facts necessary for diagnostic reasoning and therapeutic intervention (Tauber, 1999). The study of, say, works of literature, or anthropological writings may provide the material that we need for analysing the various forms of medical as well as other healing practices (Puustinen, 1999b, 2000). Finally, developments in the philosophy of medicine have revitalised philosophical enquiry into the relationship between the general (medical theory) and the particular (clinical phenomena). Such developments have revived the question of the nature of practical reasoning, which is the very substance of everyday medical practice (Toulmin, 1982). All of this requires the use of historical, linguistic, anthropological and also semiotic methods. Therefore, if we consider the medical consultation to be the constitutional basis for medicine, then the humanities are both theoretically and methodologically intrinsic to the development of medical theory.

Conclusions

The questions of how the doctor interprets the patient's complaints, how signs are produced and selected, and how diagnosis and treatment are eventually decided on during a clinical encounter have not been satisfactorily answered as yet. The vagueness of the interrelationships between biomedical knowledge and medical practice still appears to be a fundamental theoretical gap in modern medicine (Paul, 1998).

The medical consultation has been offered as a basis on which the development of the theory of medicine should be built. The clinical interaction may be seen as a form of human activity that is based not on what doctors and patients *do*, but on the *interrelationship* between the two participants. This activity is what constitutes medicine. Approaching medicine as a human activity that is undertaken in pursuit of healing may offer us new possibilities for developing a philosophy of medicine in which medicine stands as a discipline in its own right.

References

Baer E (1988) *Medical Semiotics*. University Press of America, Lantham.

Cassel E (1984) *The Place of Humanities in Medicine*. Hastings Center of Society, Ethics and the Life Sciences, New York.

Cassel E (1991) *The Nature of Suffering and the Goals of Medicine*. Oxford University Press, New York.

Cassel E (1997) *Doctoring: the nature of primary care medicine*. Oxford University Press, New York.

Engel G (1978) The need for a new medical model: a challenge for biomedicine. *Science*. **4286**: 129–35.

Engel G (1992) How much longer must medicine's science be bound by a seventeenth-century world view? *Psychother Psychosom*. **57**: 3–16.

Engel L (1997) From biomedical to biopsychosocial. Being scientific in the human domain. *Psychosomatics*. **38**: 521–8.

Evans M (1998) *Pictures of the Patient: medicine, science and humanities*. In: Occasional Paper 76. The Royal College of General Practitioners, London.

Green J and Britten N (1998) Qualitative research and evidence based medicine. *British Medical Journal*. **316**: 1230–2.

Korsch B, Putnam S, Frankel R and Roter D (1995) An overview of research on medical interviewing. In: M Lipkin, S Putnam and A Lazare (eds) *The Medical Interview. Clinical care, education and research*. Springer-Verlag, New York, pp. 475–81.

Leiman M and Stiles W (2002) Integration of theory: methodological issues. In: P Nolan and I Sävstad-Nolan (eds) *Object Relations and Integrative Psychotherapy. Tradition and innovation in theory and practice*. Whurr Publishers, London, pp. 68–79.

Lloyd GER (ed.) (1983) *Hippocratic Writings*. Penguin Books, Harmondsworth, pp. 145–7.

Mayr E (1998) *This is Biology: the science of the living world*. Belknap Press/Harvard University Press, Cambridge, MA.

Paul N (1998) Incurable suffering from the 'Liatus theoreticus'? Some epistemological problems in modern medicine and the clinical relevance of philosophy of medicine. *Theoretical Medicine and Bioethics*. **19**: 229–51.

Pellegrino ED (1983) The healing relationship: the architectonics of clinical medicine. In: E Shelp Earl (ed.) *The Clinical Encounter. The moral fabric of the patient–doctor relationship*. D Reidel Publishing Company, Dordrecht, pp. 153–72.

Pellegrino E and Thomasma D (1981) *A Philosophical Basis of Medical Practice*. Oxford University Press, New York.

Pendleton D (1986) Doctor–patient communication: a review. In: D Pendleton and J Hasler (eds) *Doctor–Patient Communication*. Academic Press, London, pp. 5–53.

Puustinen R (1999a) Bakhtin's philosophy and medical practice – toward a semiotic theory of doctor–patient interaction. *Med Health Care Philos*. **2**: 275–81.

Puustinen R (1999b) Abdu'l Qader – a portrait of a Saudi healer. *Suomen Antropologi*. **4**: 131–41.

Puustinen R (2000) Voices to be heard – the many positions of a doctor in Anton Chekhov's short story 'A Case History'. *J Med Ethics: Med Humanities*. **26**: 37–42.

Simpson M *et al*. (1991) Doctor–patient communication: The Toronto consensus statement. *British Medical Journal*. **316**: 1230–2.

Tauber A (1999) *Confessions of a Medicine Man. An essay in popular philosophy*. The MIT Press, Cambridge, MA.

Toulmin S (1982) How medicine saved the life of ethics. *Perspectives in Biology and Medicine*. **25**: 736–50.

Toulmin S (1993) Knowledge and art in practice of medicine: clinical judgement and historical reconstruction. In: C Delkeskam-Hayes and MA Gardell Cutter (eds) *Science, Technology and the Art of Medicine*. Kluwer Academic Publishers, Dordrecht, pp. 231–49.

Viljanen A-M (1999) A culture of psychiatry and culture in psychiatry: pathologizing gypsy culture. *Suomen Antropologi*. **4**: 114–30.

Wulff H, Pedersen S and Rosenberg R (1990) *Philosophy of Medicine: An introduction*. Blackwell Scientific Publications, Oxford.

The registrar crossed the corridor to the doctors' changing room, looking for a hot drink. The coffee-machine was empty.

'It's broken,' said the Accident-and-Emergency consultant, who came into the room at that moment. 'You'll have to go to the canteen if you want coffee – and don't be too choosy. Here – what happened to your thumb? Looks impressively useless'.

'I cut it in theatre.'

'Well now, I'm sorry to hear that – but not during surgery? No blood contact with the patient, I trust?'

'Well, actually, yes, there was.'

'You've been to the lab, then? No? Look, off you go now. Better to be safe than sorry. How bad was it? Just a flesh wound, or something deeper?'

'No, nothing deeper, by the look of it.'

'You'll know soon enough.'

'I suppose you can't really be sure, though, in surgery.'

'Actually, you can't be sure anywhere in medicine.'

You're certain that's what's wrong?
The problem of knowledge in medicine

Pentti Alanen

- What disease do I have?
- How do you know that?
- What are my chances of recovery?
- Is this operation safe in my case?
- Are you sure?
- Please explain why you are so sure.

People usually visit doctors because they believe (or know, or suspect) that something is wrong with their health, and because they believe (or know, or suspect, or hope) that doctors can help them to answer the questions listed above. Doctors have, at least in theory, the best opportunity of establishing the patient's state of health. A basic assumption in healthcare is that it is necessary to know the correct diagnosis in order to be able to select a relevant treatment.

The concept of evidence-based medicine (EBM) is today vividly discussed in medicine. Many practitioners seem to accept this renewed formulation of one of the Hippocratic principles. What then is this evidence that we are all asking for? The problem is that virtually none of the most enthusiastic proponents of EBM can satisfactorily define what evidence is. If a patient asks for a thorough explanation of their condition, the physician can sometimes feel quite helpless. On the basis of his education and clinical experience, he may know *that* the suggested treatment should lead to a highly probable recovery (or at least offer the best prospects of recovery), but he seldom knows in detail *why* the treatment helps. He also encounters the tension between general treatment principles resembling natural laws and explanations on an individual level. The suggested treatment has been shown to help in most cases, but how can you convince yourself and your patient that this will also be the result now? Can patients be explained as individual cases of universal laws of nature, or is individual history a totally different field of enquiry? Can we predict human destiny in a similar way to predictions in ideal experiments? Is experimental science an ideal for all areas of human enquiry?

Truth and evidence

Because the patient's life and health can be, and often are, in the hands of the doctor, the doctor is responsible both for finding the correct diagnosis and for choosing the right treatment. The problem of truth arises here in a very concrete way in everyday practice. What is the relationship between the concept of evidence and the concept of truth? There is fairly widespread agreement that no satisfactory theory of truth exists at present. Discussions of this topic are ongoing all the time in the philosophical literature. Philosophers find it hard to avoid the feeling that the discussion about EBM is superficial, conducted without any real attempt to analyse the concept of evidence in detail.

The commonest theories of truth are the *consensus, pragmatic, coherence* and *correspondence theories of truth*.

- The *consensus* theory holds that a hypothesis is true if everyone accepts that the theory is true.
- The *pragmatic* theory holds that a hypothesis can be tested by following its predictions. If the result in practice is the same as that predicted by the hypothesis, the hypothesis is correct.
- The *coherence* theory holds that a hypothesis is true if its statements fit well with other statements in the field, like the pieces of a puzzle.
- The *correspondence* theory holds that a linguistic statement gives a correct picture of the empirical world (i.e. that it corresponds to reality).

From the viewpoint of medicine, the theories of coherence and correspondence seem intuitively to belong more to the world of theoretical science, and the theories of consensus and pragmatics seem to belong more to the clinical world. However, the difference between theoretical knowledge and clinical practice is not an entirely clear one. Michael Polanyi declared that *a diagnosis is a hypothesis* and *the treatment is a test of its validity* (Schwartz, 1974).

Unfortunately, in clinical practice we cannot simply test our diagnoses by applying treatment in order to see whether the diagnosis is correct. There are two main reasons for this. First, for obvious ethical reasons, we can't experiment with patients simply for curiosity's sake – we have to be as sure as possible before deciding on their treatment. Secondly, many experts in the theory of science have put forward the charge that empirical research cannot offer decisive proofs *for* a theory, but can only disprove a theory. If this is correct, then it is treatment failures rather than treatment successes that have the greater power of demonstration – proving, for instance, the falsity of a claim that 'such-and-such a treatment always works'. For these reasons, experimental science (which is often seen as an ideal method in the search for truth) does not give us clear practical guidance for making clinical decisions.

Most people would agree that the *consensus theory of truth* – whereby truth stems from what people agree upon – is too simple. It is possible for people to agree just because they are all wrong in the same way! However, truth is not a matter of what we choose, nor is it based on voting. The only reason why it is possible for people to disagree is that they accept some common basis of rules for argument and discourse. If the opinion of one participant in a dispute implies nothing for the truth of what his opponent says, then there really would be no point in disputing, and nothing to dispute about.

However, although an agreement is clearly not a valid demonstration of truth, in real life, social pressure makes it very difficult to resist the general opinion, even when one can show that public opinion is wrong. Usually it takes an innocent child to declare freely that the emperor has no clothes. There are some notorious examples in the history of medicine (or for that matter in the history of science in general) which show what happens to dissidents. In medicine, the most famous case might be that of Semmelweiss, who discovered and demonstrated why the mortality figures on his hospital's labour and maternity wards were so high, and subsequently lost his job. These types of examples are sometimes used to defend a 'romantic' picture of science, but they should not be automatically accepted as a general rule. We may misunderstand geniuses, but not every eccentric person who is misunderstood is a genius.

Necessary and sufficient criteria for truth

The pragmatic theory of truth is the view that we ordinarily follow, almost automatically. If we believe in a theory and follow its guidelines in clinical work, and if everything is going well and our prognoses are correct, then we become increasingly convinced that the theory is correct. However, it is quite easy to see why particular examples might not present decisive evidence for our theory. It is entirely possible that although our diagnosis is wrong, the treatment we offer also happens to work for the disease that our patient actually suffers from. Sometimes the patient can get better without any treatment at all (or even despite it). The famous Goodman's paradox shows why a simple agreement between theory and practice falls short of guaranteeing the truth (even though it is a necessary part of truth that theory and practice do indeed agree). Let us assume that all of the emeralds unearthed so far have been green. We can then generalise as follows:

All emeralds are green.

In order to study this generalisation, imagine that we then formulate an additional hypothesis:

All emeralds are red, but change their colour to green five minutes before they are unearthed.

We can immediately see that all of our observations are also in perfect agreement with the second hypothesis. Despite this, no one is likely to claim that our observations provide any support for *this* hypothesis. In view of this, perhaps the empirical evidence also fails to provide support for the first hypothesis, that all emeralds are green – something more is needed. Of course, for the hypothesis to be correct it is *necessary* that our observations are consistent with it. However, it is not enough – it is not *sufficient*.

As the well-known philosopher of science Sir Karl Popper has repeatedly stated, proof and disproof are not symmetrical cases – they do not work in the same way. Clinical experience never gives absolute certainty to our diagnoses – it never conclusively proves them. However, experience can *disprove* our diagnoses. In real life, it is much easier to try to find a counter-example (and to disprove a hypothesis, just one counter-example is all that we will need) than it is to demonstrate that all the instances of a certain kind are similar. I shall now explain why this is so.

A generalised statement such as 'All emeralds are green' seems to mean 'Emerald a_1 *and* emerald a_2 *and* a_3, *and*, etc. are green'. In elementary logic, a *conjunction* of simple sentences is true if and only if *all* of the contributing simple sentences are true. Therefore a proponent of the theory that all emeralds are green has to show that every single emerald given to him is green. A sceptic will say, on the contrary, 'Emerald a_1 *or* emerald a_2 *or* a_3 *or*, etc. is not green'. In elementary logic, a *disjunction* of simple sentences is true even if only one of the contributing simple sentences is true. One is enough! A *single* exception to the rule 'all emeralds are green' is enough to show that the rule must be wrong. This is why good counter-examples are so powerful in science. They can reveal contradictions between our theories and reality. These contradictions then have to be resolved – usually by modifying and sometimes by abandoning our theories – if we want those theories to help us to understand the phenomena being studied.

Thus, good scientific studies are *critical* by nature. They are good theories if they give us the greatest possible chance of revealing counter-examples (if any exist) of what the theory claims. The task of a scientist is thus not to try to prove their theories, but to take the position of an opponent, testing their own theories to destruction, and trying to disprove them by trying to find counter-examples. If after a fair attempt has been made to find them, none are found, then we can at least temporarily accept our theory as a guiding principle. However, we cannot be absolutely sure – the theory is tolerated *provisionally*.

For many psychological, professional and social reasons, a scientist is often reluctant to reject his or her favourite theories. The scientist may find it difficult to think of a study that is capable of disclosing counter-examples. Therefore, a better idea is to have two competing schools with different, contradictory theories about the same topics, each trying to find errors in their opponents' theories. This is part of the reason why freedom of thought and freedom of open criticism are so necessary to science.

However, we need to put this still more carefully. Experience can reveal a contradiction between theory and observation, but might still be unable to locate the error in detail. The counter-example (or alternatively the counter-hypothesis) could itself also be wrong, or misleading. Our emerald example is so crude that everyone can immediately see that the second hypothesis is incorrect. In real life, mistaken hypotheses are usually not so obviously wrong. A more elaborate hypothesis, such as 'All emeralds found no deeper than 5000 metres from the surface are green, but others located deeper are violet' already *seems* to have a scientific structure. Significantly, it puts limitations on our generalisation about green emeralds. These limitations happen to be spurious, or mistaken – but the attempt to set *some* limitations is reasonable, because such limitations are very likely to exist. Similarly, many practical guidelines in healthcare may have restrictions even though we do not (yet) know them. Despite this, we have to live with generalisations and their limitations. If we demanded absolute certainty before acting, then all healthcare would have to be stopped. For instance, it would be totally impossible to vaccinate newborn babies. How could we ever be sure that no problems would arise in the babies whom we vaccinated?

A single observation of a green emerald deeper than 5000 metres below the surface would be enough to disprove the second hypothesis. However, consider again the hypothesis that: 'All emeralds are red until five minutes before being unearthed, at which point they become, and remain, green'. This point actually cannot be settled by observation – there are no colour observations that *can* be made with regard to emeralds before they are unearthed!

Thus if observations alone cannot help us to decide between this hypothesis and our first hypothesis (emeralds are simply green), why are we so sure that the first one is the better hypothesis? The explanation is that, apart from itself being consistent with empirical observation, the first theory also meets other important criteria for a scientific theory. It is more objective because it is not restricted by what the observer can observe. It is also simpler because it does not assume that emeralds can guess what time they will be unearthed! Furthermore, this first hypothesis is empirically testable, whereas the second one is not. In this way it fulfils the paramount criterion for a genuinely scientific hypothesis, as suggested by Sir Karl Popper.

Even so, the most important reason for our intuitive acceptance of the first hypothesis is that it fits logically with our *paradigms* – that is, the way in which we see the world.

Empirical generalisations and natural laws

Empirical experience can give us generalisations of the following type:

All solid spheres of gold (Au) have a diameter of less than one mile.

As far as we know, there are no exceptions to this generalisation. Even so, the generalisation is contingent fact, not a law of nature. It may be that in the entire universe there is simply not enough gold for a mile-diameter sphere, but we know of no law of nature that prohibits in principle the existence of such a ball. By contrast, consider the following sentence:

All solid spheres of uranium$_{235}$ isotope have a diameter of less than one mile.

This does indeed seem to be a consequence of a natural law. The existence of such a ball seems to be impossible because uranium$_{235}$ is radioactive, so a chain reaction would destroy such a ball immediately. The difference between empirical generalisations and scientific theories is that the generalisations declare *that*, whereas scientific theories explain *why*. A well-known example on a chess grid helps to illustrate this difference further. This example has recently been used by Simon Singh (1997) to demonstrate the difference between natural sciences and mathematics in his famous book describing how Andrew Wiles solved Fermat's great theorem in 1993. This famous theorem had remained unsolved after 350 years of unsuccessful attempts. Let us assume that we have a normal chessboard with 64 squares (32 black ones and 32 white ones), and 32 'domino' pieces such that each of these pieces is equal to two squares on the grid. One can see that it is possible to cover all of the squares with the domino pieces without breaking them. We then remove two squares, A1 and H8, from the opposite corners of the board and put one domino piece away. Is it now possible to cover all of the remaining 62 squares with the 31 domino pieces without breaking them?

A natural scientist would perhaps start with empirical experimentations. After a few hundred futile attempts, he would *believe* that there is no solution, but he could not be absolutely sure because the number of different possibilities is enormous. In this particular example it would actually be possible to go through all of the alternatives in the long run, because although the number is enormous, it is still definite. However, the situation is different in biological sciences, where typically we are considering indefinitely many future cases involving indefinitely many future organisms. (So, for example, how could we find out whether a current medication is suitable for babies who will be born in the future?)

A theoretician analyses the situation in a different way. If he observes that one domino piece necessarily covers one white square and one black square, and we have cut off two squares with the same colour, he can go on by concluding that 30 first domino pieces would necessarily cover 60 squares (30 white ones and 30 black ones). The remaining two squares would be of the same colour. Therefore it is impossible to cover all of the squares. Now we know *why*. We can also enlarge our theory for boards with other numbers of squares, other shapes of board, and for other numbers of squares to be removed. Thus we can see the logical power of an explanatory theory over empirical experience. It would now be quite simple to create a diagnostic test to find out which cases are in principle solvable and which cases are futile, at least using the present method. Whenever two squares of the same colour are removed, there is no solution. Whenever two squares of different colours are removed, there is always a solution.

The *physical* situation would naturally also be the same for boards with squares that were all of the same colour, but in that case it would be very difficult to distinguish the solvable from the unsolvable cases because visually they would look very similar to one another. A clinician often encounters this kind of situation. Patients look alike, but a given treatment helps only some of them – we just do not know whom or why. Thus our knowledge, based on empirical experience, is expressed in sentences such as the following:

> *After surgical treatment, the survival rate after 5 years is 60% for this subtype of that disease.*

... or something similar. A suitable diagnostic test would solve this problem if it could reveal the basic underlying difference between the solvable and unsolvable cases, but this requires us to have theoretically understood the nature of the particular disease. Therefore the task for a scientist is to try to change our empirical generalisations (which show *that*) into explanatory theories (which show *why*). Interestingly, Aristotle used medicine as an example to illustrate this distinction, pointing out the differences between physicians with experience but no understanding, theoreticians with understanding but no experience, and true experts with both knowledge and experience (1990, *Metaphysics* I, 981a–981b).

Guiding principles

We have not yet completely finished with our chessboard example. The 'absolute' mathematical proof given by Singh is in fact mistaken. It *is* possible to cover all of the squares even in the case where the excluded squares are of the same colour. We first cover all of the squares except two on the opposite sides of the board, and then bend the board to form a cylinder so that the two uncovered squares are located side by side and put the last piece (itself also suitably bent) in its place. We can now see that our 'absolute' proof was valid only for two-dimensional boards. We can also see that our study design was based on unconscious prejudices. Because we had assumed without further consideration that only two-dimensional cases were relevant, we had constructed our research equipment in such a way that it was not possible even to address three-dimensional objects.

This example demonstrates what is wrong with the *coherence theory of truth*. The logic of our theory was correct inside our background theory. The pieces of the puzzle had a logically perfect fit, or coherence, with the other pieces, but the internal coherence of the theory did not rescue it from the external criticism that the background *paradigm* itself was incorrect – it did not fit the real world.

The example also demonstrates one important difference between epidemiology and experimental science. The advantage of experimental research over epidemiological research is that the study subject can be artificially forced to present examples for observation, while only naturally occurring cases can be observed in epidemiological research. However, the selection of experimental procedure and equipment also sets constraints that do not apply in epidemiology. Experiments are powerful, but they are directed according to underlying hypotheses. Nature can produce examples beyond the imagination of the experimentalist. These examples can be observed provided that preconceived ideas do not blind the epidemiologist. One day, an open-minded clinician actually could meet a 'cylindrical chess board' in real life – something which is impossible for the experimentalist. It was suggested recently that night-work could increase women's risk of developing breast cancer. The suggested explanatory model was based on changes in hormonal secretion associated with changes in luminosity. An interesting detail was added in the news report. An open-minded researcher obtained his idea for the study from the clinical observation that blind women seem to have a smaller risk of breast cancer than their sighted peers. This observation served as a starting point for the hypothesis.

This type of situation is often encountered in the history of medicine. Diseases have been classified in a particular way, which guides treatment, but if a new horizon is opened, other possible risk factors and classification options become available. A contemporary case is that of *Helicobacter* (Le Fanu, 2000, pp. 147–56). After the identification of *Helicobacter* in the stomach wall, gastritis and peptic ulcers were understood as infectious diseases (this development was as recent as 1983), and consequently their therapy underwent clear changes. Recent studies have further refined the role of *Helicobacter* in the aetiology of stomach diseases, but the important point is that however our understanding of these diseases develops in the future, an infection model is now available and will remain so. Again, it is the details of the story that are interesting and which demonstrate the influence of earlier paradigms. Initially, researchers were unable to grow *Helicobacter*. After 34 futile trials, the next attempt was unintentionally interrupted by an Easter holiday. As a result, the three additional incubation days led to the growth of the bacterium. Earlier theory and experience had guided the study design and the organised attempts to grow the bacteria within a shorter time period. A similar although less well-known story is connected with the discovery of penicillin by Fleming in 1928. In this case, too, the first attempts to grow penicillin were unsuccessful, but the explanation for this was only realised in the 1960s. An exceptionally cold 9-day period occurred in London at exactly the time when the first observations were made, and the particular subtype in question did require a low temperature to grow. Again, routine but mistaken assumptions in study design spoiled the trials (Le Fanu, 2000).

These examples demonstrate the power of the background theory in study design. In 1935, a Polish physician, Ludwik Fleck, published *Genesis and Development of a Scientific Fact*, in which he described how new facts are identified in science. Fleck's idea can be illustrated by the problem of over-matching in case–control trials. For rare diseases with a long exposure time, it is useful to apply case–control study design. For that setting, patients (cases) who have the disease are compared with healthy controls, usually matched according to age and gender (no one would compare, say, a 60-year-old female patient with a 30-year-old healthy male control in order to identify differences in their exposure history). However, age and gender are not the only possible factors to be matched for comparability. One could make the cases and controls as similar as possible according to height, weight, hair colour, education, occupation, residence, working circumstances, income, family structure, number of siblings, diet, physical condition, hobbies, etc.

Now an interesting problem arises from the fact that the more variables that are included in the matching, the greater is the risk that our result will be biased in such a way that we underestimate the role of the true causal factors. The explanation for this is simple. The more similar the groups are, the more likely it is that both groups have lived in similar circumstances and, as a result, have been exposed in a similar way to the true causative factors. Since our controls are disease-free subjects, it follows that they must have unusual resistance to the exposure. They have remained healthy despite that exposure. We are comparing them with 'normal', 'typical' subjects who have been unable to resist the risk factor in question. This involves us, unwittingly, in a biased comparison which leads to the conclusion that the studied risk factor is less important – or even that it is not a risk factor at all.

Now we are caught between two extremes. If we do not match cases with controls at all, we shall not obtain any information. If we match them completely and in every respect, we shall obtain a wrong result. What, then, is the correct degree of matching? Obviously the answer is that one should not match any of the operative variables that actually play a part in causing the disease in question. Equally obvious, this in turn means that to design the study perfectly, we have to know which are the causative factors beforehand, in order to exclude those factors from the matching. However, the whole study is organised in order to find out those very causative factors! We seem to be caught in a circle.

Fleck has stated the following:

> all really valuable experiments ... are ... uncertain, incomplete, and unique. And when experiments become certain, precise, and reproducible at any time, they are no longer necessary for research purposes proper, but function only for demonstration or *ad hoc* determinations.

If a research experiment were well defined, it would be altogether unnecessary to perform it. For the experimental arrangements to be well defined, the outcome must be known in advance; otherwise the procedure cannot be limited and purposeful.

... the number of possible determinations of characteristics depends upon the habits of thought of the given scientific discipline; that is, it already contains directional assumptions.

Direct perception of form requires being experienced in the relevant field of thought.

(Fleck, 1979, pp. 85–92)

Thus there is a clear circle of understanding and interpretation (a 'hermeneutic circle') in the natural sciences: 'One has to understand in order to be able to understand'. However, it is important to realise that this is not a vicious circle but a fruitful circle. We all realise that it is impossible to ask *anything* before one understands *something*. The father of phenomenological philosophy, Edmund Husserl, said that all of our scientific problems have been pre-scientifically organised in our everyday, ordinary lives. The task of a scientist is not to abandon all of his prejudices in order to have an 'objective' attitude towards his problems, but rather to be as conscious as possible about his own commitments, so that he can see the role of his background theories and so avoid wrongly generalising from them.

In order to be able to launch a study, an examination or a diagnostic procedure, one has to have a working hypothesis, and to accept some starting point in order to be able to pose relevant questions. It is natural that the starting point and the working hypotheses can include mistaken assumptions about the nature of the phenomena under study, simply by virtue of being based on earlier knowledge of the topic. This can lead to mistaken or insensitive selection of the experimental equipment, or to other types of methodological problems, thereby preventing our understanding of the phenomena under study. It may then take several futile attempted experiments before we begin to suspect that something is wrong in our assumptions. If we are fortunate, something will then dawn on us and we will change direction towards an answer. Afterwards, we can easily see how our thinking was constrained by too narrow an understanding of the situation. If we draw three circles on a piece of paper, O O O, and ask an innocent participant to add two lines to the picture to get a dog, most people start drawing long lines to obtain a *picture* of a dog. However, instead of a picture, two simple short lines can be added to produce letters, creating the *word* 'dog'.

In this way we can see how our background assumptions drive our research enquiries. If we see the phenomenon under study from the correct point of view, we select our equipment and measuring apparatus in such a way that none of the hidden assumptions of our methods conflict with the nature of the subject that we are studying. As long as everything is running well, we have no reason to suspect our methodology. However, our equipment is also a part of nature, obeying nature's rules. We cannot assume that we have (unconsciously) correctly understood all of the properties of the world before making our observations. If some new observation contradicts our unspoken assumptions about the way in which the equipment works, then our research programme will be in difficulties. We can only proceed if we succeed in identifying the reason for the contradiction.

The example of the bent (and twisted!) 'cylindrical' chessboard shows that it can be possible to refute even supposedly absolute mathematical proofs by empirical counter-examples that reveal the structural limitations of the proof. This example also explains why absolute proofs may be impossible even in those cases where we think that we know the truth of the matter. A logical proof is indeed capable of showing why the theoretical assumptions behind the study design (including any that are hidden or unstated) are consistent with the observations arising from the study, and it is capable of unifying assumptions and observations within the same theoretical framework. However, it cannot prove that the theoretical assumptions behind the study are themselves correct, regardless of how perfect the fit may be between the observations and our underlying theoretical paradigm.

Truth-as-correspondence *vs.* 'seeing in the light of paradigms'

We are left with the *correspondence theory of truth*. According to this theory, a sentence such as 'The book is on the table' is true if it gives a correct *picture* of the world (i.e. in this simple case, the sentence is true if we can see that in fact the book is on the table!). In the real world of experience we have all kinds of objects, and in language we have names for those objects. In terms of the correspondence theory of truth, a scientific theory is correct if it gives a correct picture of the world. However, there is a basic problem with this theory.

Look again at the previous paragraph. We did not in fact compare our sentence with the empirical world. Instead, we compared two written expressions, namely a sentence in quotation marks, and the same words outside quotation marks. Perhaps we could try to eliminate this problem by pointing with a finger at the physical situation, at the same time holding up a piece of paper on which we had written, 'As you can see, the book is on the table'. Does any problem remain now?

The trouble is that the procedure of pointing is only successful if the observer already understands what 'pointing', 'table', and 'book' mean and which types of objects can be identified as books or tables. In other words, the observer must already have mastered some part of the language, and must already have a (loosely) theoretical understanding of the world which defines objects as books, tables, etc. Only *within* such a theory is it possible to apply the correspondence theory of truth. Thus a picture theory of language cannot be fundamental; there always has to be something deeper behind it. From this we can see that a theory of truth which is itself based on picture theory cannot be fundamental.

Let us clarify this idea with a medical example. Imagine that a doctor has reason to suspect that her patient has cancer. In order to be sure, she takes a biopsy, which is sent to a qualified pathologist who examines the sample under a microscope. Based on professional experience, he gives his diagnosis, it proves to be correct, the doctor treats the patient accordingly, and his life is saved. If a layman looks at the same biopsy sample under a microscope, from the optical or physiological point of view he will see exactly the same as the pathologist, but he cannot make a diagnosis because from the point of view of understanding or interpreting, he cannot see what the pathologist can see at all. A layman does not know what the shapes, sizes, colour and amount of cells and nuclei, etc. *mean* with regard to the health status of the patient because he does not have a specific theory.

In our everyday life we also see the world through theories, but we are too accustomed to our theoretical ways of seeing the world to recognise the role of our paradigms. It is one of the most commonly accepted ideas in modern theories of knowledge that all empirical observations are theory-laden. (In hermeneutic philosophy, the favourite expression is 'something is seen as something'.) As a result, it is not possible to compare language and the world without relying on some theoretical assumptions about the world, and these assumptions give us our (typically unconscious) criteria for what is true and what is false. The point is that we are still comparing *two interpretations* (i.e. language and theoretical assumptions), and we are not comparing one interpretation of the world with the empirical world itself – we simply do not have direct, unmediated access to the world. Theory and language always stand between us and the world. As a result, the correspondence theory of truth can never carry out its claimed task.

Treatment, prevention and aetiology

Now there is a further aspect to be discussed. We can ask 'Why does this treatment help?', and we can also ask 'Why does this factor increase the probability of developing a particular disease?', but the answers to these two questions need not be logically connected – treatment and aetiology are not necessarily dependent on each other. Surgical operations or medication do not necessarily aim to eliminate the causative factors. They may aim to eliminate the diseases as such, or they may simply aim to achieve the palliation of symptoms. An operation to remove cancerous tissue does not even try to eliminate the causes of the cancer – it merely removes one result of those causes. The operation itself is based on the assumption that in many cases no new cancers will appear, even if the causative factors are not eliminated. The same is true for many cases of medication. Pain or inflammation are treated in the hope that the organism itself will be able to recover if the burden of the disease is eliminated, even if only temporarily.

The situation with regard to prevention is different. Disease cannot be actively prevented without breaking the causal chain at some practicable point. Therefore prevention is more theoretically based than treatment, and it calls for an understanding of the causes of disease. The pragmatic theory of truth may therefore play a different role in everyday practice to the role that it plays in aetiological research.

Experimental science is often seen as the 'gold standard' for all research. In experiments, one strives to regulate and control the assumed causal factors in order to make it possible to draw conclusions from what happens. However, experiments are not – and should not be – free from preconceived ideas and assumptions. As the above example of the chessboard demonstrates, the whole study design, the selection of relevant equipment, the calibration of measuring instruments, etc. are based on assumptions about the nature of the phenomena under study. Without them it would be impossible to conduct any empirical studies at all. The more aware the researcher is of his or her theoretical assumptions, the better he or she is able to see their limitations and capacities, and the better he or she is also able to change them, at least in principle.

Assumptions underlying experimental science

Now let us consider a comparison between the sciences and the humanities. Patients are individual people with their own backgrounds and their own 'histories', who are looking for a personal encounter with appropriate healthcare professionals. Patients are urgently asking for a prognosis ('What will happen to me?'). However, exact predictions seem to work well only in the natural sciences and not in the behavioural sciences, or in history. There are various theories that try to encompass this difference between physics and history, saying for instance that history is just too complicated compared, for example, with weather forecasts (which are not particularly successful either, we might think). Some theories have tried to reduce the subject matter of the humanities to descriptions in physics, which is taken to be at a more advanced stage of development. However, this reduction also leads to a 'two-dimensional' restricted form of explanation. Consider the following sentences:

About five thousand million years ago, the Earth was a hot ball. No life was present on its surface. Life is now present. Therefore life can be explained in terms of the material phenomena described by physics.

It seems difficult to avoid the given conclusion, since the preceding sentences seem to be true. Consider, then, the following sentence:

All pirots are carylating in an elatic way.

Is this sentence-like line of letters also true? One is inclined to say that there is no real question of the truth or falsity of this supposed sentence, because it means nothing. Some meaning is required for there to be any analysis of the sentence's truth. However, the same holds for the (true) sentences about the early stages of the Earth.

Meaning implies a language, which in turn (for us, at any rate) implies human culture. In our terms, the *question* of the truth or falsity of any meaningful sentences implies the concerns and enquiries of human beings. Thus the concerns of human beings as subjects, participants and observers are intrinsic to objective science, and cannot be separated from it – language and the world are interwoven.

In the Aristotelian tradition, the behaviour of inanimate objects was understood in similar terms to the behaviour of human beings – that is, as purposeful and aiming at certain ends. According to this theory, the movements of physical objects were classified as natural (i.e. towards their goal), or unnatural (i.e. forced or constrained). Forced movements did not reveal the properties of nature, because in those cases the objects under study lacked the opportunity to move naturally, or in accordance with nature. Thus one of the most important rules for an Aristotelian scientist was the following: *Do not disturb natural phenomena if you want to find out the principles that they obey.* As a result, passive observations were possible, but experimental science, which disturbed the natural state of phenomena, was impossible.

After the Galilean revolution in science, it became clear that the movements of inanimate objects cannot be explained by comparing them with human behaviour. Physical movements in nature have no purposes or aims, but follow 'blind', unchanging, natural laws. The triumph of modern natural sciences was thus established. Unfortunately, this tradition also resulted in a theory with only one explanatory principle – this time based on an idea opposite to that which underlies Aristotelian theory. Researchers tried (and many still do) to explain human behaviour in the same way as they explained the phenomena of physics – that is, in terms of 'blind', unchanging natural laws.

As a result, the way was left open for experimentation, and this became one of the most important and decisive steps towards modern science. A researcher could now formulate exact questions and use them to interrogate Nature – which was obliged to answer if the question was formulated correctly. Nature had no alternative to its standard way of functioning in these controlled, experimental circumstances, and thus the observer could register Nature's answers. One of the basic rules in this form of experimentation is the following: *You cannot disturb the study setting if you want to know how Nature really behaves.* Experimental results are simply not credible if the conditions of the experiment are altered, disturbed or tampered with.

Bearing this principle in mind, imagine the attempt to predict human behaviour. Suppose that the investigator in a particular study predicts that all subjects sitting in the room will stand up after five seconds. The prediction is uttered, five seconds elapse, and no one stands up. Now the investigator can still maintain that his prediction has not been falsified because (no doubt for reasons of their own), having heard his prediction, the subjects then simply decided to interfere with the study. If they had not behaved so as to disrupt the study, the investigator could maintain, his prediction would have succeeded.

The point of this example is that predictions in the natural sciences are made not with respect to actual, historical, particular time (in which the context is crucial), but with respect to a hypothetical, generalised, theoretical and universal time scale (from which all local, particular context has been rigorously abstracted). Thus it is a profound mistake to try to extend the ability of the natural sciences to make physical predictions into the realm of real, historical, context-bound behaviour and events. The predictive powers of the natural sciences are based precisely on the exclusion of human behaviour from their experiments – as we said, you cannot disturb the study setting if you want to know how Nature really behaves. It is a straightforward methodological error to try to generalise from the results of predictive natural sciences to intentional human behaviour (which of course inherently involves the very aspect which had to be excluded from natural science experiments).

Ernst Mayr (1997) is one of the very few scientists who have strongly emphasised this clear difference between logical predictions and historical predictions. For example, Darwinian theory helps us to understand how a species may have developed through non-directed variations and natural selection, but this theory does not predict which types of species will survive in the future. Perhaps one of the main differences between today's physics and biology is that biology turns out to be a partly 'historical' science, in this sense of having to take context into account, whereas physics is understood as a non-historical science in pursuit of unchanging natural laws.

Concluding remarks

If predictions in biology differ from predictions in physics, then so too prognoses in healthcare differ from the hypothetical predictions of physics, which do not concern real, calendar, historical time. However, this is only one side of the picture. Whenever we make use of our knowledge of physics, chemistry or pharmacology, we have to apply their general principles in a specific historical situation and to an individual case. Thus the real-life applications of the relevant sciences are tied into the historical time scale, and all of our predictions and prognoses concern calendar time.

In practice, we rarely achieve absolute certainty in clinical predictions. The reasons for this concern not only the difference between physical and historical predictions, and the variation and complexity of biological phenomena, but also the fact that, for ethical reasons, we cannot simply stop our clinical work in order to wait for the emergence of 'final' or conclusive data before we take our clinical decisions. Patients would suffer and die while we waited. Thus, regardless of the unavailability of conclusive data, we just have to rely on accumulated clinical experience, empirical generalisations, lists of contraindications, etc. We can never be absolutely sure of what we do, but we have to accept our personal responsibility to do our best in the absence of final truths, for both theoretical and practical reasons. Consequently, the ethical responsibility of a clinician is always bound up with his knowledge and his historical situation.

References

Aristotle (1947) *Metaphysics I* (transl. GC Armstrong). Heinemann: Loeb Classical Library, London. 981a–981b.

Fleck (1979) *Genesis and Development of a Scientific Fact*. The University of Chicago Press, Chicago.

Le Fanu J (2000) *The Rise and Fall of Modern Medicine*. Carroll & Graf, New York.

Mayr E (1997) *This is Biology: the science of the living world*. Harvard University Press, Cambridge, MA.

Singh S (1997) *Fermat's Enigma. The epic quest to solve the world's greatest mathematical problem*. Fourth Estate, London.

Schwartz F (ed.) (1974) *Scientific Thought and Social Reality: Essays by Michael Polanyi*. International Universities Press Inc., New York.

The registrar went to the canteen, retrieved a cup of coffee from the machine and bought a roll. The hospital chaplain was talking to another junior doctor at the only available table.

'What happened, then?', asked the other doctor. The registrar described the accident.

'A heavy night's drinking?'

'Since you ask, I'd been on call all night. I've slept two hours in as many days.' He sighed. 'I should never have started that appendix.'

'I dare say you're blaming yourself?', the chaplain asked.

'No. Well ... a bit,' muttered the registrar.

'It's what happens,' said the chaplain. 'You over-work, and then you feel guilty about not spending time with the family. You under-work, and then you feel guilty about not giving your all to the patient and to the clinical team. You make mistakes and then feel guilty. Not to mention when you get ill. There's a lot of guilt around in hospital work.'

The other junior doctor winked ('beware the priest') and left.

This cancer's my punishment, isn't it?
Guilt, shame and medicine

William Stempsey

Introduction

Mr Black, who is 50 years old, has smoked two packets of cigarettes a day for more than 30 years. Although he has had a chronic 'smoker's cough' and periodic respiratory infections requiring antibiotic therapy, he has never seriously considered the effects of smoking on his health. He now notices some tinges of blood in the sputum he coughs up. X-rays reveal a mass in his lung, and a biopsy shows that he has a primary lung carcinoma. He asks 'Why did this have to happen to me?'.

Mr White, who is also 50 years old, has never smoked. He has carefully watched his diet and exercised regularly. However, a routine physical examination, which included a colonoscopy, reveals a moderately advanced carcinoma. He asks 'What did I do? Why has this happened to me?'.

Baby Blue, only 6 years old, develops acute lymphoblastic leukaemia. This disease is now routinely put into long remissions with chemotherapy. Talk of cures has even become commonplace. Yet Blue's case is different. Chemotherapy fails to effect a remission, and she is close to death. Her parents ask 'Why has this happened? She does not deserve this!'.

In all three cases the same question is asked. When we get sick, it seems natural to wonder why we have become ill. In Mr Black's case, it is tempting to offer a quick and easy answer: 'You got lung cancer because you inhaled a known carcinogen daily, almost constantly, for more than 30 years.' The other two cases are not so likely to evoke such a glib answer.

The more 'scientifically-minded' physician might simply say that we do not know why these people got sick, but one day research will tell us. However, it does not take much common sense to realise that such answers miss the point. The question 'Why did I get sick?' is often not seeking a scientific explanation – it is seeking a philosophical explanation. When people get sick, they have a tendency to ask questions that reflect wonder about their existential predicament. Why must I die? Why must I die now? Why must I die in this way? Why did I get sick? These are the big questions, and they are philosophical questions.

As Aristotle observed in his *Metaphysics*, philosophy begins in wonder. Such questions are expressions of the wonder that naturally arises in us when we are confronted with the many mysteries that life presents. There are no easy answers to such questions. Ultimately, there is no single answer to these existential questions that will satisfy everyone. One of my teachers in medical school once said 'Some people get sick and some don't.' This is undoubtedly true, and it shows a wisdom that is deeper than one notices at first glance. The answer raises more philosophical questions about the meaning of life and how best to respond to what life presents us with. There are many other fascinating answers as well, and that is what makes the study of philosophy so captivating. Physicians need to recognise the importance of such questions to patients, and at least be supportive of their patients' quest for answers.

However, in asking the 'Why?' questions about illness, people are some-times asking a particular kind of philosophical question. We might call this type of question a moral question. The question here is 'Did I myself do something to cause my illness? Should I be held responsible for doing it?'. It is natural for people to wonder whether they have done something to cause their own illness. In the case of the smoker, it is tempting to blame the victim. Yet the causation of any disease is a complex one, and such blame may be simplistic. After all, other people smoke for a lifetime and never seem to suffer any ill effects. Yet even in cases where there is no obvious explanation as to what has led to the person's illness, it is natural to wonder whether one might still be to blame. The patient has a tendency to wonder whether some behaviour has, unbeknownst to him or even to anyone in the scientific community, contributed to the illness. Patients are often heard to ask 'Was it something that I did, or something that I failed to do?'. Speculation is likely to preoccupy a patient ('if only I had taken a daily vitamin pill,' 'If only I had listened to my friend and practised yoga,' 'If only I hadn't eaten so much fried food').

The experience of illness brings many emotions, of which guilt and shame may be among the most prominent. Patients may feel guilty (rightly or wrongly) about having brought about their own illness. They may feel ashamed that they are ill. The encounter with the physician also provides ample opportunity for the patient to feel shame about his or her body and bodily functions.

Physicians are prone to experiencing feelings of guilt and shame as well. The physician who treats Baby Blue may well experience guilt about not having cured a patient with a disease that is normally cured. The physician might wonder 'Did I do something wrong in this particular case?'. This may lead to guilt and shame even though the physician gave the best possible care. Then again physicians, being only human, make mistakes. Unfortunately, they are sometimes actually guilty of causing harm or even death. Feelings of guilt and shame are inevitable in such cases.

Sometimes a question about whether a mistake was made is not really a moral question at all, but a larger existential question. Physicians encounter incurable illnesses all the time, and are powerless to do anything to save their patients. They must, if they are thoughtful, wonder about the larger meaning-of-life questions that are raised by their work. This can lead to feelings of guilt and shame, too. Physicians may also experience shame about their inability to answer the existential questions that patients raise.

Guilt and shame are complex emotions. They are related, and are often confused. It is sometimes difficult to say exactly what they are and how they differ. Physicians must be able to recognise these emotions in their patients if they are truly to be healers. They must also be able to recognise these emotions in themselves if they are to function effectively and not be crippled by them. Finally, they must recognise that they have the power to induce guilt and shame in their patients. They must know how this happens and whether or not it is proper in the many different activities that constitute medical practice. What follows is an attempt to clarify just what guilt and shame are, and the role that these emotions play in the experience of illness and the practice of medicine.

Guilt and shame

Our first task will be to clarify exactly what we mean when we talk about guilt and shame. They are well known to almost everyone, yet it is not easy to differentiate them in a precise way. What does seem clear, however, is that guilt and shame are emotions.

Emotions are complex phenomena, and as such they can be classified in many ways. Philosophical analysis of emotions tries to offer explanations of their nature and their genesis, and to clarify any relationships that exist between them.

Guilt and shame are included, along with pride and humiliation, in what Gabriele Taylor (1985) has called the 'emotions of self-assessment'.

Guilt and shame are feelings that we have about ourselves – about who we are and also about what we do. We often do not make precise distinctions when we think about these types of feelings. We are as likely to say that we are ashamed of something that we did as to say that we feel guilty about what we did. We might also say that we feel embarrassed. However, all of these feelings indicate a process of self-assessment about our character or our actions, or both.

The emotions of self-assessment provide us with a means of evaluating ourselves. Evaluation is a comparison of how things are with how things ought to be. We evaluate things all the time. Physicians evaluate health and disease in their patients, and in this evaluation they use relatively objective standards. Critics evaluate works of art, and in this evaluation they use some objective standards, but they use their own subjective aesthetic standards to a higher degree. The type of evaluation that is associated with guilt and shame falls into the moral realm. Guilt and shame are indicators of the goodness and badness that we attribute to ourselves. These emotions are concerned with the moral status not only of our actions, but also of our very selves – our character.

For this reason, guilt and shame are usually recognised as moral concepts. In general, we say that someone is guilty when that person has broken some law or violated some code of behaviour that is accepted by society. Moral guilt has the same type of structure as legal guilt. One becomes guilty by violating some law, whether it is civil or moral. We can be guilty of breaking a law without knowing it or admitting it. Feeling guilty, on the other hand, seems to be a separate issue. We might rightly feel guilty (when we truly have broken some law), but we might also feel guilty without justification (when no law has been violated). Shame, in contrast, seems to depend on our feeling ashamed. We cannot feel ashamed without knowing about it. In contrast to the situation with guilt, we cannot *be* ashamed without knowing it.

It is sometimes said by anthropologists that modern Western society has become a society of guilt. The contrast is drawn between our modern society and the society of the ancient Greeks, which is said to have emphasised shame. This is not to say that the Greeks did not recognise failure to obey law. It is just that their ethics emphasised virtues of character, especially such virtues as courage and justice. Emphasising personal character rather than individual actions puts more of an emphasis on shame than on guilt.

To be shamed is to be discovered to be lacking some aspect of what a proper sort of character should have. Shame is associated with being seen acting inappropriately or in the wrong circumstances by an audience that matters to the individual. In Homer's *Odyssey*, Odysseus is ashamed to be seen by certain people when he is crying. This would seem to that audience to be a manifestation of a lack of courage, a defect of character. The function of shame is to prevent one from doing such things. Shame should prevent people from doing things that bring dishonour to them.

Shame is particularly associated with nakedness. The Greek word for genitals, *aidoia*, is derived from the word for shame, *aidōs*. If we are caught naked unexpectedly, our natural reaction is to cover ourselves, especially what we call our 'private parts.' In such situations we are likely to feel ashamed. Of course, similar feelings occur in other situations that are unrelated to nakedness.

Shame is not just a matter of being seen. It is also a matter of being seen by an observer whose opinions matter to us. We are not ashamed of criticism from someone whose views we do not respect. Furthermore, actual observation by others need not occur. Remember that shame is an emotion of self-evaluation. One can feel ashamed by merely imagining acting in a shameful manner in the presence of some person or persons whom one deems to be important in the relevant way. Even so, as Bernard Williams (1993) has pointed out, feeling shame at being naked would be merely a pathological fear if it only involved being found out by a purely imaginary observer and never involved any actual observation by others. We can feel shame when we are alone, but we are ashamed because our self-evaluation tells us that whatever is the cause of our shame would be disapproved of by the relevant kind of audience, whether that audience is present or not.

This point is illustrated by the story of the ring of Gyges in Plato's *Republic*. The story is told by Socrates to argue against the claim that justice is nothing more than seeking one's own advantage and that people would do anything to further that advantage if they thought they could get away with it. From deep in the earth, Gyges recovers a ring with a remarkable property. When Gyges wears the ring in the normal way, nothing unusual ocurs. However, when he turns the ring on his finger so that the collet faces toward the inner part of his hand, he becomes invisible. Equipped with this ring, he can do anything that he wants without being found out. He seduces the queen, kills the king, and takes over the kingdom as his own.

Socrates' use of the story is effective because the reader with a proper moral character will immediately recognise that right conduct does not merely depend on whether one will be found out or not. Gyges has no shame. The internalised audience that should prevent him from carrying out his heinous acts is absent. The person with a properly developed sense of shame would not do such things, even though they could not possibly be seen by those who would disapprove of the actions.

Williams argues that although the Greeks had no direct equivalent of what we call guilt, their sense of shame must include more than we narrowly conceive of as shame today. In Homer's writings, the reaction to someone who has acted in a way that shame should have prevented is called *nemesis*. This reaction to such an action might be shock, contempt, rage or indignation. This notion of *nemesis*, as we shall see presently, involves responses that we would consider proper to both guilt and shame. According to Williams, shame and guilt both involve an internalised figure. In the case of shame, the figure is a watcher or a witness. In the case of guilt, the internalised figure is a victim or an enforcer.

Although the Greeks seemed to conflate what we call shame and guilt, the fact that we have two separate words for these emotions means that there probably is an important difference between them, at least on a psychological level. The kind of thing that produces guilt in an individual is an act or omission that typically provokes in others a sense of anger, resentment or indignation. The proper response to one who is guilty is to demand reparation and perhaps to inflict punishment. On the other hand, the kind of thing that produces shame in an individual is something that provokes contempt, derision or avoidance in others. Shame also differs from guilt in another important respect. Something that induces shame might be an act or omission, but it might equally well be some personal physical defect over which one has no control. Thus shame is not grounds for demanding reparation or punishment. Shame just makes one want to disappear. At the time of writing, a memorable set of television advertisements for an airline is being shown on television in the USA. These advertisements show people doing various things that we would not consider to be moral or legal transgressions, but which are nonetheless major causes of embarrassment. In one advertisement, a man is in a church attending a wedding and talking to the person next to him about the bride. Suddenly the organ stops playing and the conversation is heard by the entire congregation. The ad ends by showing an aeroplane along with the slogan, 'Want to get away?'. This is a good example of shame caused by being overtly found out by a group considered by the individual to matter. The man wants to get away – to disappear from sight. However, he has no fear of being punished or carried off to jail, and therefore, there is no guilt.

Bearing in mind these general considerations about shame and guilt, let us consider shame and guilt separately in a little more depth so that we can reach a better understanding of the role that they play in medical practice.

Shame

'Shame cultures' are distinguished from 'guilt cultures' in that public esteem is held as the highest good in shame cultures. Public esteem for the individual depends on how the individual is judged according to some code that expresses the society's values. To violate this code is to ruin one's reputation and lose the esteem of other members of the society. To be regarded badly is the greatest evil in a shame culture. From a Western liberal perspective, we might well ask if a person really deserves the honour or dishonour bestowed by society. After all, one's reputation is not always reflective of what the inner person is like. However, such distinctions do not make sense in a shame culture.

This is not to say that there is no distinction between the outer and inner person in shame cultures. The ancient Greeks certainly did recognise this distinction. However, there is a key difference. Modern individualists tend to say that if one has done no wrong, then one should still be proud of oneself, even if one is scorned by society. This would not be possible in a shame culture. When one's reputation is lost in a shame culture, one's value is lost in the eyes of all members of the society, and this includes one's own eyes. With regard to shame, there is no distinction between public and private. Self-assessment depends on public assessment.

In Jean-Paul Sartre's *Being and Nothingness* (1956), a man makes a vulgar gesture. Only afterwards does he realise that he has been observed. This realisation then makes him look at himself through the eyes of the observer. From this other vantage point, the man realises that his gesture is vulgar, and he feels shame. The man accepts the judgement of the observer and admits that he is acting in a vulgar way. It is not just that the man realises that he has done something unacceptable. The new realisation changes his attitude toward himself – he feels degraded and shamed. Only by seeing himself through the eyes of another does the man feel shame (Emad, 1972).

However, this is not to say that an actual observer is required to feel shame. As Sartre's example suggests, one individual can take on two different roles – that of actor and that of observer. An artist can be critical of their own work. This criticism does not require any audience. The artist might just be ashamed of their work. However, the judgement involves taking an alternative viewpoint of the critic, apart from the viewpoint of the creator.

However, shame requires more than simple judgement about the work of art. It also involves a judgement about the way in which the artist views him- or herself. An artist who feels true shame feels shame not only about the work of art, but about him- or herself. But why should this be? One bad work of art does not necessarily make a bad artist. Something more seems to be necessary. The way in which the artist perceives him- or herself to be seen by the critic seems to be a crucial element. Audiences, or imagined audiences, have different characteristics. The artist may perceive the audience to be friendly and accepting, extremely critical, sophisticated or naive. The crucial point about shame is that one's assessment of oneself depends on a relationship with an audience. We may be quite willing to sing at parties among accepting friends, but most of us would feel ashamed to inflict our performance on paying customers in a concert hall.

The philosopher Max Scheler has provided an interesting example (Scheler, 1957). A woman who has been posing nude for an artist for some time suddenly comes to feel shame when she realises that the artist no longer regards her as a model, but as an object of sexual interest. The model becomes aware of a changed point of view on the part of her observer. Her relationship with the artist has changed. Formerly, the relationship was an impersonal one. Now it is personal, and the model sees her exposure as improper in the new (or newly imagined) circumstances. The feeling of improper exposure leads her to feel shame. The model need not take upon herself the artist's point of view. In this case, in fact, the model feels shame because she is observed by an improper audience, and not at all the one that sets the standards of shame and honour. The person feeling shame judges herself adversely. She does not see her judgement as depending on the judgement of the audience. Thinking of herself as being seen in a certain way has made her feel inferior to what she had felt or hoped to feel. Thus shame is what Gabriele Taylor calls the 'emotion of self-protection'.

The origins of shame in ancient shame cultures are evident enough. Shame arises from membership of an honour group. When one violates the honour code of the group, one feels shame. Again it is important to realise that shame is not simply the censure of the group – it is also something that is felt by the individual. This is because the identity of the individual is so importantly a function of membership of the group. It would not be quite accurate to say that individuals are secondary to society in such shame cultures, for there is a robust individual sense of self in such cultures. However, individuals in shame cultures see themselves formed by and dependent on society in a way that those in modern cultures do not. Modern Western societies are able to understand the concept of an individual defending personal beliefs without shame in the midst of a disapproving society. However, this would not happen in a shame culture. While people in modern Western societies do not live in shame cultures, they are nonetheless familiar with feelings of shame.

A modern account of shame is given by contemporary philosopher John Rawls (1971), who notes that shame is a feeling that comes with the experience of injury to one's self-respect. Self-respect includes a sense of one's own value, the conviction that one's life plan is worth pursuing, and the confidence that one has the abilities necessary to carry out that life plan. Shame is intimately connected with our own person and also with those on whom we depend for confirmation of our own sense of personal worth. Shame is painful because it is the loss of a primary good.

Rawls distinguishes between two different types of shame (Rawls, 1971). Natural shame arises from injury to our self-esteem as a result of not having or failing to exercise certain excellences. It is our plan of life that determines what we feel ashamed of, and so shame is influenced both by our aspirations and by the people with whom we want to associate. One may feel ashamed of one's appearance, or of some other personal characteristic. However, a simple lack is not enough to induce natural shame. The lack must be associated with one's aspirations or one's view of how others perceive one. A person with no musical ability does not feel shame so long as he or she has no aspirations to become a musician. However, a surgeon who lacks the dexterity to suture skin neatly may well feel shame.

The second type of shame in Rawls' account is moral shame. When one adopts a life plan, one embraces various virtues. These virtues are desirable both to the individuals and to those other people with whom he or she associates. Actions that manifest a lack of these virtues are then likely to be the source of shame. Rawls notes that both moral shame and guilt might arise from such a situation, but that moral shame and guilt do not have the same explanation. He asks us to consider the example of someone who cheats or gives in to cowardice and then feels both guilty and ashamed. The person feels guilty because the action was contrary to their sense of right and justice. They expect others to be resentful, and they fear the possibility of reprisal. Moral shame, on the other hand, arises because the person has failed to achieve the good of 'self-command' and has been found unworthy by the people on whom they depend for confirmation of their sense of self-worth. The person's behaviour has provided evidence of the lack of moral excellence that the person prizes. With guilt, we focus on the violation of the just claims of others. With moral shame, we focus on the loss of self-esteem and our inability to carry out our life plans.

Guilt

Having considered shame, let us now turn to a consideration of guilt. Gabriele Taylor explains that guilt, unlike shame, is a legal concept (Taylor, 1985). Guilt results from breaking a law, whether that law is of human or divine origin. The action that gives rise to guilt makes one liable to punishment or, if proper repentance occurs, forgiveness.

We may be guilty without feeling guilty, and we may feel guilty without actually being guilty of having transgressed any law. To feel guilty, we must accept that we have done something forbidden and also accept the authority of whoever forbids that action. If we do not accept the authority of the law-giver, then we might not feel guilty even though we *are* guilty of violating the law. Of course, we can also feel false guilt when we think that we have violated a law but in fact have not done so.

Taylor observes that the notion of an authority plays a role in guilt that is analogous to the role that an audience plays in shame. As with the audience in the case of shame, the authority in the case of guilt is not always clearly identifiable. The violation of law that provokes guilt feelings may simply be the violation of some taboo. Taboos exert great authority in the minds of many, even when there is no actual authority present to regulate the behaviour involved.

To be guilty is to deserve punishment for one's transgression of the law. To feel guilty is to think that one is deserving of punishment. Both guilt and punishment focus on a particular act that is deemed to be punishable. Thus guilt is localisable in a way in which shame is not. Feelings of guilt are concerned with particular actions, whereas feelings of shame are concerned with the type of person one is. Because feelings of guilt are connected with a particular action, it makes sense to think about repayment for that action in a way that would not make sense for shame. If I am guilty of an action that harms another, I owe it to that person to 'make up' for what I have done with some kind of repayment, or at least by suffering some form of punishment. I seek to be forgiven. With shame, on the other hand, there need be no particular action to forgive. There may be nothing for which to offer repayment or be punished.

It is possible to feel guilty for some action, but not to feel that performing that action has changed the essence of who one is as a person. For example, if I park my car and fail to put the proper fee into the parking meter, I may be (and feel) guilty of breaking the law. I feel that it is justified that I should receive a parking ticket and pay a fine. I may feel no shame so long as I do not make illegal parking a habitual practice. However, if I habitually park illegally and ignore the parking tickets, this behaviour says something about my character. I am the kind of person who scoffs at the law, and may well feel ashamed of this.

Furthermore, guilt is related to my taking action in a way that shame may not be. If I am guilty of breaking some rule, it is because I consciously take an action that goes against some law or presumed law. When I break a rule unknowingly or by accident, I am either excused or my guilt is mitigated. If my car hits a hidden patch of ice and slides into another car, causing damage, I am not guilty of malicious destruction of property in the way that I would be if I had deliberately rammed another car. Shame, on the other hand, may be related to circumstances that are completely outside my control. I may be ashamed of the shape of my nose, or some other feature of my body, and I have no control over such matters. Neither punishment nor forgiveness is appropriate in this case. While paying a parking fine will serve to remove guilt, no penalty will relieve the shame that I feel about my body.

Guilt and shame in medical practice

Guilt and shame, in these many different manifestations, are commonly felt by both patients and physicians, but especially by patients, in their everyday encounters. Studying guilt and shame can help physicians to act more effectively as healers, and it can also help physicians to cope with the stresses that are inherent in medical practice. For patients – and even physicians become patients at some time or another – the study of guilt and shame can help them to come to terms with illness, to accept responsibility for health maintenance, and to obtain relief from false guilt about their role in bringing illness upon themselves. Let us then look more closely at how guilt and shame may have an impact on both physicians and patients.

Physician guilt

Doctors are only human – they make mistakes. Although a few of these mistakes might actually be violations of civil or moral law, most of them *are* simply mistakes. Guilt is certainly a factor when laws are broken, but physicians may also feel guilt about their unintended mistakes.

Feelings of guilt are warranted when they result from actual transgressions of law (true guilt). Feelings of guilt may also be completely unwarranted (false guilt), even though the feelings are quite real. Whether guilt is warranted or not depends on a complex set of factors.

Consider the example of a patient who dies during surgery for a ruptured spleen. Does the surgeon incur guilt for the death? The answer to that question depends on many things. We first want to know why the patient died. What was the cause of death? It would make a great deal of difference if the patient was already near death from blood loss when the surgery started, or if the death was the result of the surgeon cutting a major artery during surgery. This question is further complicated by the difficulty of deciding exactly what the cause of death is in any case. We often do not consider the complexity of this issue of causation. Any death is the result of many contributory factors, many of which are never noticed. When a respirator is removed from a patient and the patient dies, is the cause of death the removal of the respirator or the underlying disease that makes it impossible for the patient to breathe? It is not easy to answer this question. Different answers have led people to take different positions on the ethics of removing life support. It is difficult to conclude that a physician incurs guilt for a particular action when that action is only one of many factors that contribute to an adverse event. Determining whether the guilt in such cases is true guilt is one of the major questions of medical ethics. However, the point here is that physicians are liable to feel guilty in the event of any bad outcome. Further analysis of the case can help the physician to deal with these feelings in an appropriate way.

Another complex situation that has a tendency to be guilt-provoking is the true ethical dilemma. An ethical dilemma is a case in which one is forced to make a choice and all of the possible options seem to be morally wrong. In the well-known Tarasoff case in Berkeley, California, a patient told his psychotherapist that he was going to kill a particular woman. The therapist faced a dilemma. Should he warn the intended victim, thereby breaking the time-honoured rule of confidentiality in the doctor–patient relationship? Or should he keep the confidence and risk the murder of an innocent woman? In such dilemmas, the bad outcomes have to be balanced and the lesser evil chosen. However, the fact remains that in making a choice in the circumstances of a true dilemma, one is liable to feel guilty irrespective of what one does. Medicine is full of such decisions. Every medical treatment, no matter how simple or common it may be, has potential side-effects. Physicians must always balance risks and benefits when recommending treatments. This sets the stage for guilt feelings, because bad outcomes do occur, even when the bad outcome seemed to be a remote possibility and worth the risk.

Physician shame

Physicians can, of course, feel shame about any aspect of their lives. This shame might negatively influence their practice of medicine. Here, however, we shall only consider physician shame that arises within the context of medical practice.

Any time when a physician does not live up to the behavioural standards of the medical profession, that physician is likely to feel shame. A physician may be ostracised by his or her peer group for any number of valid or invalid reasons. Unfortunately, personal conflicts can lead to the exclusion of perfectly competent individuals from professional groups. Although this may be ethically unacceptable, it can nevertheless be a source of shame for the excluded physician.

In cases where physicians are not capable of doing something that they ought to be able to do, or that they believe they ought to be able to do, they may feel shame. This might be related to incompetence, but it is more likely to result from simple human limitations. For example, if a physician in training fails to hear a heart murmur, and a more experienced physician points out that the younger physician 'missed the diagnosis', the younger doctor is likely to feel shame. Physicians are assumed to have the physical diagnosis skills that are necessary to detect heart murmurs, and to miss an important physical finding is likely to make a physician question his or her own competence. Professional competence is in part a question of what kind of physician the individual is, and not just a question of one wrong act – a faulty diagnosis. Thus it is a matter of shame. Examples such as this are numerous.

Patient guilt

Patients may experience guilt feelings in many situations. As with Mr Black, the smoker who developed lung cancer, people engage in behaviours that are known contributors to disease. These people may feel guilt about bringing on their own illness. Even individuals such as Mr White, who have not engaged in any behaviour that is known to cause disease, may feel guilt. Such people may feel that they have done something to bring on their illness, even though they do not know exactly what it was. Rene Dubos traces back to Hippocrates the idea that people have a good chance of escaping disease if only they live reasonably. He argues that 'the concept that disease results from the failure to behave according to natural laws accounts in part for the fact that illness is more often associated with a sense of guilt than are other misfortunes' (Dubos, 1987). It seems that patients have a 'subconscious sense of responsibility' for their fate. Physicians can play an important reassuring role in their relationships with patients who have such feelings.

On the other hand, physicians can also reinforce guilt, whether that guilt is true or false. Physicians, as well as other people, can sometimes have a tendency to blame the victims of disease for their own predicament. They may be inclined to think 'If only you had stopped smoking, as I told you to, you would not have got this cancer,' or 'if only you had exercised more and been more careful with your diet, you would not have had this heart attack.' Physicians may also want to blame patients for not seeking treatment soon enough. For instance, a woman may notice a breast lump but not seek treatment until the cancer has spread or even ulcerated the skin. Patients may sometimes be afraid to seek treatment even when they know that they are ill. They may also deny that their symptoms and signs of disease are really significant. Physicians need to remember that such patients are suffering greatly and need support and care. Even if blame seems appropriate, it will not help these patients. Physicians may also want to blame their patients for not responding to therapy in the way that is expected. This may actually result from failing to carry out the doctor's orders exactly, but it is also the case that sometimes people just do not respond to treatments that almost always work. Again, even in those cases where blame for failure to follow the physician's recommendations seems appropriate, it will not help patients.

There are many reasons for resisting the temptation to blame victims of disease. In many cases, the behaviour that has contributed to a particular disease was engaged in before the connection with the disease was even suspected. It would be foolish to blame older adults who develop skin cancer because they were overexposed to the sun during childhood. No such association between sun exposure and skin cancer was known during their childhood. Furthermore, as we have already seen, the causation of disease is complex and not completely understood for many (if not most) conditions. Singling out one behaviour as justifying guilt about disease causation is just too simplistic. As Richard Gunderman points out, the physician's objective is not to determine who is at fault in producing a disease, but rather to treat disease, relieve suffering and promote health (Gunderman, 2000). The nature of medical practice is rooted in the fact that patients suffer from disease and that physicians often have the ability to relieve that suffering. Although medicine has an essential moral dimension, physicians are not trained to be moral judges. It is not their role to punish their suffering patients further – even those who may truly be guilty of contributing to their own suffering.

Sometimes patients' guilt might lead them to want to accept their illness as a just punishment for their misdeeds. As a result, they might refuse necessary treatment. This is especially true of diseases that result from engaging in some form of socially scorned behaviour. For example, a patient with AIDS may view his disease as a punishment for homosexual behaviour, and feel a need to atone for his 'sin'. Peter Marzuk argues that by readily acceding to such a patient's refusal of care, in the name of respecting patient autonomy, the physician may 'unwittingly and improperly ally himself with the masochistic elements of the patient's character' (Marzuk, 1985). Sometimes a physician needs to resort to a limited type of paternalism so that a patient's guilt does not lead to self-harm.

These are not easy judgements to make, and there are no facile rules that physicians can employ in order to make them. Individuals may refuse treatment even when that refusal will lead to their harm or even death. Ascertaining whether a patient is competent enough to make such decisions is an art that is not easily learned. This limited paternalism, although it ought to be regarded as a last resort, may sometimes be justified in order to preserve a patient's true autonomy.

Patient shame

The nature of medical practice demands that patients sometimes be naked before their physicians and, as we have seen, shame is particularly associated with nakedness. Medical practice thus provides ample opportunity for patients to feel shame. Although nakedness alone is enough to provoke feelings of shame, other factors are also likely to provoke such feelings. The patient's encounter with the physician in the context of the physical examination may reveal physical defects that are a source of shame for the patient. For example, one patient may be ashamed of having a club foot. Another may be ashamed of being overweight. Even in the absence of overt physical defects, patients may feel shame about revealing some aspect their bodies, even something that is quite normal. Illness can also give rise to unpleasant bodily odours from faeces, urine or vomiting. In addition, illness may have prevented the patient from attending to everyday matters of personal hygiene. All of these things are potential sources of shame.

Physicians always ask patients to relate the history of their illness. In telling their story, patients may well feel shame about various issues. As we have seen, they may feel guilty about certain things that they have done and that they perceive to be related to their illness. Such guilt about a particular action may lead to feelings of shame about being the kind of person who would do such a thing (Hartmann, 1984).

Illness can be debilitating. It can rob a person of the self-sufficiency to which that person is accustomed. A patient may feel shame about being unable to carry out the activities of daily life that are taken for granted by most of us. When patients enter a hospital, they often experience an upsetting loss of individuality and self-reliance. They may even feel as if they have become laboratory animals, subject to constant observation and testing.

All of this can be a serious affront to the patient's self-image, and a source of profound shame. In medicine, many things that are usually kept private must be revealed to another, often a comparative stranger. Shame is a way we have of protecting our privacy. Matters concerned with sex and excretion, in particular, have to be revealed to physicians, and these are the matters that are most strongly associated with shame.

Finally, shame can be associated with death. Carl Schneider (1977) points out that 'mortification', which means shame or humiliation, has an etymological connection with death (in Latin, *mors*). The connection between shame and wanting to disappear is related to this. Dying is the ultimate way of disappearing. We use expressions such as 'I was so ashamed that I wanted to die.' As Schneider points out, the dying person is surrounded by sources of shame – loss of control over bodily functions, the presence of tubes and catheters, child-like dependence on others, the stigma of being incurable, and the gathering of family and friends, who often feel embarrassed themselves. Death itself can even be regarded as an offence and shameful. In modern times, people seem to have lost the ability to see death as something natural. Instead, death has become something to fight and conquer. Physicians can unintentionally reinforce this feeling in their efforts to cure illness. We do not like to talk about death, and being forced to face death can bring the most profound sense of shame.

Conclusion

Medical practice is an encounter between a physician and a patient. What brings the physician and the patient together is the fact that the patient is experiencing illness. We have seen many ways in which the experience of illness can provoke guilt and shame – both for the physician and for the patient. We have examined some of the complex explanations for the sources of guilt and shame. Awareness of these matters can help physicians to be more comfortable with themselves as they attend to the needs of their patients. It can also help physicians to alleviate the suffering that patients experience as a result of their own guilt and shame.

References

Dubos R (1987) *Mirage of Health: utopias, progress, and biological change.* Rutgers University Press, New Brunswick, NJ.

Emad P (1972) Max Scheler's phenomenology of shame. *Philos Phenomen Res.* **32**: 361–70.

Gunderman R (2000) Illness as failure: blaming patients. *Hastings Center Rep.* **30**: 7–11.

Hartmann F (1984) The corporeality of shame: *Px* and *Hx* at the bedside. *J Med Philos.* **9**: 63–74.

Marzuk PM (1985) The right kind of paternalism. *NEJM.* **313**: 1474–6.

Rawls J (1971) *A Theory of Justice.* Harvard University Press, Cambridge, MA.

Sartre JP (1956) *Being and Nothingness: An essay on phenomenological ontology.* Philosophical Library, New York.

Scheler M (1957) Schriften aus dem Nachlass. In: *Gesammelte Werke.* Francke, Bern.

Schneider CD (1977) *Shame, Exposure and Privacy.* Beacon Press, Boston, MA.

Taylor G (1985) *Pride, Shame and Guilt: emotions of self-assessment.* Clarendon Press, Oxford.

Williams B (1993) *Shame and Necessity.* University of California Press, Berkeley, CA.

Now somewhat revived by the coffee, the registrar pushed open the swinging double-doors into the pathology department. The waiting-room was full. He sat on a plastic chair outside one of the clinical cubicles, within which he could hear a crowded conversation involving several voices with strong local accents. After a minute or two, a veiled female technician pulled back the curtain and ushered out three fully-veiled Muslim women. She then motioned to the doctor to enter the cubicle, and swept the curtain closed again. She took off her veil and examined the injured hand.

'Ouch, what happened to you?'

'Forget how – the question is "when". I had a blood contact with a surgical patient.'

'Right, let's check your antibodies.'

'I haven't seen you wearing a veil before.'

'Well,' explained the technician, 'in fact I do come from a Muslim family, but I don't usually wear the veil – except here at work, with some of my Muslim patients. Some of the older Muslim ladies are pretty strict about who can examine them.'

'Yes, all right, I've noticed.'

The technician put a tourniquet around the doctor's arm.

'I suppose you know this is going to sting a bit.'

'Uh-huh.'

The technician pressed the needle into a suitable vein.

'You know, some of these ladies don't want blood tests taken during holy festivals. It really strikes you, sometimes, how faith and beliefs can affect the way people approach their doctors. Or the way they use their medications.'

'I'm no longer surprised by what people do. Doesn't mean I understand it, though', the registrar responded. 'In fact, since you ask, I'm often tempted to say to my patients that medicine is just medicine, and it doesn't care what you think or what you believe. It works, or it doesn't work, and that's an end to it.'

'You could *say* it. But it wouldn't convince them. And it wouldn't really convince you, either, would it?'

'To be honest ... maybe not.'

Tao of medicine? Cultural assumptions in medical theory and practice

Shinik Kang

The world, human beings and culture

We tend to take for granted existing conventions and institutions and say that they are natural or the most advanced ones. A European or American citizen might think that a general election is the most *rational* and therefore *natural* way of choosing political representatives. However, a king or a minister of a monarchy might think a little differently. They might think that they themselves had a right and at the same time a responsibility to rule and protect their people. Someone living in the Amazon rainforest might see things differently again. They might not understand what democracy or even politics means. A Hindu guru might find all of these institutions vain. In each of these instances one's own world is collectively constructed by one's fellow people. And we call the worlds that are constructed in this way *cultures*.

We might think that Euro-American culture is superior to Amazonian or Indian cultures. We might believe that Western culture is more widely relevant than others. We might also believe that it is superior because it incorporates the concepts of human rights and egalitarianism. We could argue even further, that Western culture is superior to any others because it incorporates the concepts of rationality and individuality that are supposedly absent from other cultures. This argument could be extended by claiming that biomedicine of Western origin is superior to other local healing arts because it is based on culture-free *science*.

However, before we finalised our argument, we would have to ask a few fundamental questions. We would have to substantiate the supposition that the very notions of individualism, rationalism and science are superior to those of collectivism, intuitionism and culture. What makes these concepts superior? Is it not ethnocentric to take these concepts for granted and apply them blindly to other cultures?

To answer these questions, let us briefly examine the concept of the person and the individual. The English word 'person' originated from the Latin word *persona* meaning 'actor's mask'. Thus it meant bodily appearance rather than inner state of the person. The origin of the term 'individual' cannot be missed. It means indivisible unity, so an individual is a single person. In both cases people are independent *entities*.

However, in East Asian culture the concept of a person is concentrated not on individual persons but on relationships between them. The Chinese word denoting 'person (人間) epitomises how East Asians have ignored the independent and individualised unit of a person. Instead, when they mention the 'person', they automatically mean people in relation to each other. The first ideogram (人) depicts the form of two people leaning against each other. The second ideogram (間) simply means 'between' or 'among'. Therefore being a person immediately means being with others or having relationships in a certain situation – in other words, *being in between* or *being in the world* in the Heideggerian sense of the terms. In this chapter I shall examine how the differences in the mode of *being in the world* (culture) have influenced healing arts as they have developed. A specific culture implies not only a specific way of *seeing* the world but also a specific way of *being* in the world. Cultures are not simply ways of treating and conceptualising the same world that exists indifferently out there. They are ways of actively appropriating and interpreting the world and the people in it. The world through which a group of people has lived is not the same as it was before it had been lived through. By seeing the world in a specific way and living in the world with that specific point of view, the people of a culture create a new way of being in that world, and thus a new world itself. This process goes on and on. Therefore both culture and the world are not static, but are constantly changing. They are not entities, but processes.

Therefore when we talk about cultures we should consider not only the spatial (geographical) but also the temporal (historical) dimensions. When we talk about the culture of a specific region or a field, we should look over the entire history of the region or the field, so that the present can be correctly situated in the historical context and the future can be anticipated properly.

> There is, then, no essential medicine. No medicine that is independent of historical context.
>
> (Kleinman, 1993, p. 23)

Medicine as culture

Thus it follows that a healing art in a specific era and place represents a specific way of making sense of and dealing with illnesses in that specific era and place. Therefore medicine as we know it today is not the only kind of medicine that could ever be encountered. In other words, a healing art (medicine) should be seen through the lenses of culture and history. Historically and culturally, there have been various kinds of healing art. The biomedicine that is now considered to be the universal mode of dealing with illnesses is only one of them. Medicine's mode of existence largely depends on the mode of seeing and being in the world of illnesses. 'Medicine, then, like religion, ethnicity, and other key social institutions, is a medium through which the pluralities of social life are expressed and recreated.' (Kleinman, 1993, p. 24)

The first sentence of the English translation of *Aphorisms* in Hippocratic Writings reads as follows: 'Life is short, *science* is long; opportunity is elusive, experiment is dangerous, judgement is difficult.'[1] However in the Korean version it is translated as follows; '... *art* (藝術) is long ...'. One of the reasons why the two languages have translated the Greek word *techne* so differently is that the Greek word had a broader meaning than either science or art. The other explanation could be that the two cultures have constructed scientific and artistic conceptions of the healing art (*techne*), respectively. In the West, most people seem to believe that medicine is a science rather than an art, although there have been hot debates on the nature of medicine.

However, in East Asian healing systems, people have tended to think of medicine as an artistic and moral project rather than a scientific one. For instance, the ideogram denoting medicine (醫) was formed from components denoting different healing arts. The first part (医) depicts the state of a person who has an arrow in his or her body. The second part (殳) depicts a spear that was used to remove the arrow. The third part (酉) denotes alcohol that was used to soothe the patient. This third part has frequently been replaced by another form (巫) denoting a shaman. Thus the Chinese ideogram that is meant to translate the English word 'medicine' (醫 or 毉) has surgical, medical and spiritual components in itself.

---

[1] Lloyd GER (ed.) (1983) *Hippocratic Writings*. Penguin Books, Harmondsworth, p.206. In other versions of the translation, it is more often translated as 'art' than 'science'. What I would like to emphasise here is the fact that Koreans *never* say that science (科學) is long, whereas Europeans sometimes do.

On the other hand, the history of Western medicine shows us that there have been separate traditions of medicine and surgery.[2] We can conclude from these stories about the origin of medicine that Western biomedicine is a historical and cultural product rather than *the* one and only system for healthcare. If we locate biomedicine within a historic and cultural context, it comes to be *a* local system of healing, rather than *the* medicine.

This does not mean that we can ignore biomedicine's efficacy and strength. At any rate, biomedicine and its allied discipline public health have contributed greatly to the improvement of both length and quality of human life. We are living longer and more comfortable lives than our ancestors who were living only 100 years earlier. There is no doubt about the fact that most fatal infectious diseases have become tamed thanks to antibiotics, a notable example of which is penicillin for pneumonia. Many people with chronic renal failure who would simply have died if they had been living in the 1950s, are today living active lives thanks to technologies such as artificial kidneys and renal transplants. Moreover, biomedicine has given us further expectations – although they may be false or exaggerated – that we shall soon conquer most intractable diseases, including cancer and genetic disorders. How can we resist this sweet promise of biomedicine?

Do we then have to accept the superiority of biomedicine to traditional East Asian medicine or other healing arts? Probably we have to. But does biomedicine fit into every aspect of human life regardless of time and space? Maybe not. Let us examine the following example. Most pregnant Korean women who had given birth to a child in Europe or America complain about the way in which postpartum care is delivered. They are surprised to find European women walking outside against the wind or stepping on a cold floor after the delivery of a child. They think that joints and muscles have undergone loosening and relocation during the pregnancy and labour. Therefore they should be stabilised by lying down on a warm floor and taking a long rest while covered with a thick blanket. Otherwise, they believe, they will experience joint pain and 'cold foot and hand' for the rest of their lives. I have indeed seen many Korean women complaining of these symptoms after delivery. They usually ascribe their complaint to inappropriate postpartum care. They believe that wind and cold are prone to invade deep within women's bodies during the postpartum period. This belief system may seem bizarre, yet we can make a number of points from this observation.

This story tells us that these women still live in and through the bodies constructed by their cultural history and not through biomedicine,

---

[2]Remember that we still use the terms physician and surgeon separately.

although they are well educated. Here comes the so-called medico-cultural conflict. However, if we accept the argument that biomedicine itself has been culturally constructed, and is not the only system of knowledge, then this boils down to a culture–culture conflict. Thus it seems that we must be prepared to accept the notion of 'medicine as culture.'

Cultures in healthcare and medicine

Even so, it is a strong claim to be asked to accept, particularly perhaps when one is a medical student. Today's medicine is largely recognised as a *science*, which is dramatically distinct from *culture* in its nature. Courses in medical schools are composed mainly of sciences (i.e. anatomy, physiology, biochemistry, microbiology, pharmacology etc.) There may be courses on social sciences and humanities, too, but fewer people accept such disciplines as 'medicine proper'. For many more people, 'good medicine' is nothing more than a 'good science'. Social sciences and the humanities are claimed to be important in medicine, but only to the extent that they help medicine proper – which is science not humanities.

However, what we find in historical and cultural materials tells us quite a different story. This chapter will attempt to explore these unfamiliar scenes. This is an exercise both in becoming a stranger to what has been very familiar to us, and in becoming familiar with what has been foreign to us. We will travel through the web of time (history) and space (culture), but in order to avoid getting lost in this complex web, we need to have a guide who chooses where to visit and what to see. I shall attempt this task. However, before we get started, I have to confess that I myself have my own history and culture, and am going to guide us according to my own interest and bias. It means that this journey is not going to be a neutral one, but heavily charged with local custom and prejudice of my own. So you, the reader, will have to become acquainted with your guide first in order to profit from the journey.

Your guide is from an East Asian country, namely Korea, so what he is going to say must have a strong local accent not only phonetically but also culturally. Therefore, in order for you to get along well on this journey, you must become acquainted with his local dialect first, although his accent is not a pure one. His education has been confined mainly to science of Western origin, rather than the humanities, although he was born and raised in Korea, where traditional Asian values prevailed. So let us explore your guide's cultural background, which has influenced and formed his present attitude towards medicine.

During this journey I would like you to consider the specific and essential elements of biomedicine in comparison with another system of medicine, namely East Asian traditional medicine. I would also like you to consider some of the differences between medicines of the past and the present in the West.

The tradition of East Asian healing art

It is generally said that today's Western medicine is the direct heir of Hippocratic medicine in that both of them are based on unbiased observation of natural phenomena in illness and healing. Thus we call Hippocrates the 'Father of Western Medicine.' However, according to medical historians, even in his own era, Hippocratic natural medicine was by no means the only healing system. Most of the Greeks went to a temple to be treated by a god's hand rather than seeing a mainly itinerant doctor. The healing profession was not a unitary entity either. There were various schools, each claiming its own healing system. There were groups of empiricists, dogmatists, eclectics and sceptics, as well as advocates of temple medicine. However,, we do not give them due credit. We speak as if Hippocratic medicine was the only Greek medicine that ever existed.

We can observe exactly the same tendency when we look at ancient Chinese medicine. There had been various different types of healing system before and even after the great classical texts appeared.[3] They included oracular therapy, demonic medicine, religious healing, pragmatic drug therapy and Buddhist medicine, as well as the formally accepted 'medicine of systematic correspondence'[4] (Unschuld, 1985, p. 4). These healing systems have had an influence well into the present time, but again we do not give them due credit. We speak as if the medicine of systematic correspondence is the only medicine that was developed in China.

What then accounts for the prominence of Hippocratic medicine in the West and of the medicine of systematic correspondence in the East? Probably it arises from our tendency to neglect those healing arts that do not have systematically written documentation. However, we have increasing evidence which indicates that people freely choose among different healing arts. Both then and now, and both in the East and in the West, people sometimes disregard scholarly based medical knowledge. Even in industrialised countries, including America, ever increasing

---

[3] *Huang-ti nei-ching* (黃帝內經), which is the oldest textbook of medicine in China, seems to have been written in about the same period as the Hippocratic writings.
[4] The system of medical knowledge that is based on the *yin/yang* dualism and the Five Phases System.

numbers of people visit alternative healers more frequently than they visit licensed medical doctors. What does this phenomenon mean? Is something wrong with the scholarly based medicines? I don't think so. It is not that any of the healing systems contain decisive errors, but rather that our perspective is too narrow. We may resort to any of the healing resources available, while still tending to regard them as non-scientific and thus unreliable. We generally regard the well-documented medical systems (Hippocratic medicine, the medicine of systematic correspondence and modern biomedicine) as scientific or at least rational, whereas the poorly documented healing systems are regarded as 'mere' expressions of culture, poorly defined and elusive. Furthermore, we tend to regard biomedicine as *the* scientific medicine, and the medicines of Hippocrates and systematic correspondence as primitive or under-developed, even if they are not entirely unscientific. Both the latter are acknowledged as being important contributors to modern biomedicine, but are viewed as being highly charged with cultures of time and place.

Here science and culture are being represented as opposing poles of the human endeavour of coping with illnesses. In reality, however, we do not care whether a method is scientific or cultural so long as it works. In short, there is no reason why the healing process should be exclusively scientific or cultural. Healing art consists not only of the scholarly mode of reasoning, but also of ill-defined influences from culture. Therefore, in order for us to understand East Asian healing art properly, we need first to understand the cultural context in which is located.

The cultural background of East Asian healing art

It is by no means an easy task to summarise briefly the essence of a foreign culture, unless you have been living with the people of that culture for quite a long time. Moreover, the culture of a region or of a time period will inevitably be a mixture of various influences from both within and without. East Asian societies have not only produced their own ideas, such as Confucianism, Taoism and Shamanism, but have also assimilated foreign ideas such as Buddhism, and more recently Christianity and Marxism.

However, it is also true that in order for people in a certain place and time to engage in a healing process, they must have some core concepts concerning health and illness. Unschuld, who is a renowned medical historian of China, calls this the 'paradigmatic core' and the other concepts that constitute its periphery the 'soft coating'. In my view, Confucianism and Taoism constitute the paradigmatic core, while Buddhism and Shamanism constitute the soft coating of traditional East Asian medicine. Unfortunately, however, we do not have enough time to look around the shrines of each denomination. We must consider the paradigmatic core first and look at the soft coating only in passing.

It is generally accepted that the dominant values of East Asian societies come from Confucianism, and that any development in science – including medicine – comes from Taoism. The basic concepts regarding the nature of the universe and of humanity came from various schools of thought that originated in ancient China, but have been conflated into Confucian doctrines. Confucianism is not only a political ideology that emphasises filial piety, but also a cosmology that explains the universe and the moral way of life. The key concepts of entire East Asian culture – yin/yang dualism and the Five Phases theory – have also been incorporated into Confucian cosmology and morality. Once established, these frames of thought were widely used to explain various phenomena, indicating natural philosophy, politics, arts, sciences and medicine. These are very much flexible frames of reasoning. Each of the Five Phases (Wood, Fire, Earth, Metal and Water) has its corresponding equivalent in medicine, politics, arts, etc. For example, the Fire Phase corresponds to the heart in medicine, the colour red in fine art, and the emperor in politics. Thus heart, the colour red and the emperor, corresponding to the Fire Phase, have implications in common. Each of the Five Phases has its own implications and corresponds to a variety of phenomena. This is what Unschuld calls 'systematic correspondence'.

On the other hand, Taoism is less concerned with social and familial orders. Instead, it tries to find a way to transcend the material world. Unlike Confucian scholars, Taoist monks prefer not to participate in political processes, and they are rather hermetic and reclusive. They try to cultivate their inner world by exercising their bodies. However, the body here is not only material but also spiritual. These two are so closely interwoven that they do not have separate words for each of them. The spiritual is to be expressed through and embodied in the material, and the material is nothing more than the spiritual. They are said to have made the substance for eternal life inside their bodies. This substance is not only produced within bodies but is also to be found outside them. By producing and consuming this substance they are believed to have lived long lives. In this sense we can even say that the Taoist doctrine has medical overtones in modern terms.

Thus Confucianism and Taoism constitute the two wheels of East Asian medical concepts. Although the two doctrines seem to contradict each other, they are complementary in any actual situation. Not only lay people but also authentic scholars of medicine freely resort to these two different schools without any hesitation. Although I have portrayed the scene as if the two schools have independent sets of ideas, they have been so frequently intermingled in cultural history that it is not easy to distinguish the influence of one school from that of the other. Further additions from Buddhism and Shamanism, which I called 'soft coatings', make the scene more perplexing still. However, we should 'intuit' rather than analyse the whole situation, because the objective of this journey is to gain a new perspective in which biomedicine – not East Asian medicine – is reflected.

Healing systems

As has already been mentioned, East Asian healing art is not based on a unitary conceptual system, but is a mixture of various influences from different beliefs. However, as far as we can discern from other healing arts, such as humoral medicine and biomedicine of Western origin, there would be no problem in giving it an independent status. It will become clearer when we have finished our visit to a traditional East Asian medical clinic and an operating theatre in China where a major operation is being performed under acupuncture anaesthesia.

First, let us visit a Chinese medical clinic where a patient examination is being conducted. Suppose that we have hidden cameras and can observe every small movement in the clinic. A doctor (or preferably a healer) is sitting at a desk. A patient enters the office, and the doctor carefully observes the appearance, gait, complexion and even the clothing of the patient. The patient takes a seat alongside the doctor. From then on the doctor pays special attention to what he smells and hears. Now a conversation begins, but the doctor tends to listen rather than talk. He pays attention not only to what the patient is saying but also to how the patient says it (e.g. the tone, colour, speed and clarity or hoarseness of the voice). Meanwhile the doctor carefully examines the patient. At this time he takes a closer look at the patient's skin, especially that of the face (e.g. texture, tension, colour, humidity, etc.). Then he examines the patient's tongue. It is said that doctors can distinguish more than 30 different states of the tongue. Finally, the doctor puts his fingers on the patient's body. Special attention is paid to the pulse that is felt from the radial artery. When the doctor feels the pulse, three fingers are used. Each of the three fingers feels a different component of what seems to be the same pulse of the same radial artery. In addition, the pulse is felt at three different pressure levels (i.e. when light, medium and heavy pressure is applied to the artery). Therefore from the single action of sensing a pulse, nine different pulses can be felt. If the pulses are taken from both arms, 18 different pulses can be felt. In addition, from a single pulse no fewer than 51 types can be identified. For example, a pulse can be classified as floating, deep, shallow, tense, feeble, strong, etc.

Now the doctor has completed his examination and has obtained a considerable amount of information about the patient. However, the information thus accumulated cannot be said to be objective, because the flow of information is not unilateral but bilateral in nature. The information is not simply gathered, but is produced by exertion.

Once the examination has been completed, the active process of syndrome differentiation begins. Here the doctor mobilises the full range of his knowledge about the universe, the country to which he belonged and the weather, as well as about the human body. He tries to find reasonable explanations for those of the patient's misfortunes which are distinguished as illness. He associates the phenomena that affect the patient with the conceptual framework of yin/yang dualism and the Five Phases theory. However, not all traditional doctors use the same framework of reasoning. Some of them explain the cause of the patient's illness mainly in terms of the so-called 'Five Organ' system.[5] However, others mainly resort to an 'Illness Factor' system (wind, cold, heat, dampness, dryness, fire, the seven emotional states, etc.) or an 'Eight Rubric' system (yin/yang, exterior/interior, cold/hot and depletion/repletion). Whatever reasoning system he has employed, the doctor draws a conclusion of his own.

When the patient's syndrome has been properly differentiated, the doctor prescribes a set of herbs or treatment modalities including acupuncture, moxibustion,[6] exercise, massage or a change of lifestyle. The whole range of treatment modalities is deployed logically according to the original syndrome differentiation.

So far we have witnessed an interesting scene of East Asian healing art, but perhaps in some ways it is not so strikingly different from the Western-style doctor's office. We might discern a resemblance between the two systems because the consultation procedure is very much the same, even though the prescriptions are different. Alternatively, we might feel that the two systems differ markedly because the basic concepts for explaining illnesses are so strikingly different. I do not want to comment further here. Instead, let us visit another room where an operation is in progress.

A Western-style surgeon has diagnosed a patient as having acute

---

[5] The Liver, the Heart, the Spleen, the Lung and the Kidney, which correspond to the Five Phases (Wood, Fire, Earth, Metal and Water).

[6] The burning of moxa or other substances on the skin to treat diseases or to produce analgesia.

appendicitis, and is planning to remove the appendix surgically. An acupuncturist is called in to administer anaesthesia. She puts several needles into the patient's skin. The surgeons then begin the operation while holding a conversation with the patient. We may be astonished to find that the acupuncturist does not use any drug to anaesthetise the patient. How on earth is it possible to get rid of the severe pain of the operation by simply inserting some needles? To date no one has been able to explain scientifically how acupuncture causes anaesthesia or other healing processes, although authentic organisations such as the National Center for Complementary and Alternative Medicine (NCCAM) of the National Institutes of Health (NIH) have officially admitted the efficacy of acupuncture.

Having witnessed scenes in which the concepts and procedures of healing are so different from those of biomedicine, we might now wonder whether biomedicine is really the only effective healing system. In the next section we shall look at the Western medical tradition from an Eastern perspective, and vice versa.

The Tao of healing art

In the previous sections we have seen that there can be different types of healing art corresponding to the world view that each civilisation developed. What we could call the 'mode of existence' of medicine varied according to these different developments. In East Asian languages, the ideogram that denotes healing art (醫) rarely exists in isolation. It usually occurs with other ideograms that make the meaning more concrete and real. For example, when it occurs with the ideogram that means learning (學), it becomes a healing art as a system of understanding. When it occurs with the ideogram that means performance or skill (術), it denotes healing art being practised. When it occurs with the ideogram that means virtue (德), it denotes healing art embodied in a person. These three modes of existence constitute the Tao of healing art (醫道), which is the supreme principle for the healing profession. Tao, which literally means 'the way', is the first principle for any profession or occupation. It can be translated more fully as 'the right way everyone should follow.' For example, businessmen have the Tao of commerce, and civil servants have the Tao of civil service. However, Tao is not a doctrine or a list of admonitions, nor is it some abstract idea from which various qualities emanate. It includes not only moral principles but also the knowledge and skills that are required to bring about healing. In summary, East Asian healing art exists in three different but closely related modes, namely as a scholarship, practice and virtue.

Healing art as a system of understanding: learning *vs.* knowing

Medical science is a scholarly system for dealing with illnesses that affect human beings. It aims to determine the phenomena of health and illness properly and systematically so that people can predict what will happen. Although the purpose of medical science is the same throughout the world, the actual system of knowledge differs significantly according to time and place. This difference arises from the different cultural assumptions that each civilisation has developed.

The word that denotes academic activities in East Asian societies literally means 'asking and learning' (學問), which is then further divided into science and humanities. Etymologically, the word that denotes science (科學) meant 'learning by classification', and the word that denotes humanities (人文) meant 'the patterns of humankind'. Traditional East Asians tended to think in terms of interaction between the knower and the known, rather than in terms of unvarying entities to be understood objectively and in isolation. On the other hand, the Western tradition of understanding emphasises 'the known' rather than 'the knower'. This difference in basic attitude towards understanding in general has produced striking differences in the medical systems that each has developed. The most striking distinction between the two medical systems can be seen in the ways in which they represent human bodies.

If you look at the sculptures and paintings of ancient Greece and those of ancient China, you will find that each of the two civilisations had its own concept of the body that is manifested through the artistic works. Figures in Greek sculptures are usually naked with prominent muscles, whereas those in East Asian sculptures are usually wearing clothes and have no discernible muscles. In a textbook of traditional East Asian medicine we find neither prominent muscles nor details of body parts. Rather we find abstract lines of meridians running through the surface of the body, and acupoints on which acupuncture needles would be inserted, none of which is actually visible on the body at all. This contrasting emphasis that is seen in works of art shows, I believe, how each tradition has made sense of the body. East Asians have tended to see and emphasise the inner state of the body and the interconnections between the parts, while the Greeks have tended to see the visible parts of the body that bring about actual movement. These different assumptions about the body will have resulted in strikingly different systems of medicine.

However, this generalisation does not seem to be applicable when we examine the medieval history of the West. From after the fall of the

Roman Empire until the Renaissance, the body was regarded as a microcosmos which embodies the Providence of God or the universal order. Following Hippocratic and Galenic doctrine, the body was visualised as a vessel containing four basic humours. The harmonious coexistence of these four humours constituted health. The correspondence between astrological constellations and body parts was also a powerful tool for explaining health and illness. This dynamic and cosmological concept of the body began to decline once Renaissance anatomists such as Leonardo da Vinci and Andreas Vesalius actually opened up the body and sketched every part of it. From then on, the body was visualised as a structure composed of muscles, vessels, nerves and bones, rather than as a container of humours. As we can see in the famous drawings by Vesalius, the body resumed actual *forms and structures* that were important in Graeco-Roman art but were lost during medieval times. Vesalius was a pioneer of modern biomedicine in the sense that he was the first to see the body not within the framework of an abstract metaphysical idea but from a detached observational perspective. This disinterested gaze at the body is believed to be the foundation of scientific medicine. From that time onward, anatomy has been regarded as the science that truly represents the body – necessarily and irreplaceably. This devotion to the true representation of the real body has been the driving force behind medical science. However, if we compare Vesalius' drawings with the modern textbooks of anatomy, we can certainly detect the difference between the two.

First, in Vesalian drawings, human subjects have their own postures and complexions, although they must be drawn from dead and sundered bodies. For example, the skeletal man is even *thinking* about something while leaning against a table. The musclular man is an athlete engaging in active exercise, although all of the skin has been stripped off. In modern textbooks of anatomy we find hardly any vividness of this kind. We can find more details of body parts, but we never find the context in which the owner of the body has been situated. What we have lost from Vesalian anatomy is the life and context of the person.

Secondly, in Vesalian anatomy we find mistakes that anyone can easily discern. For example, if we look at the drawing entitled 'female reproductive organ' we might think that the title must have been misprinted, because it certainly seems to be a male reproductive organ. However, in fact this is not the case at all. Vesalius seems to have thought that the female reproductive organ should be the exact negative template of the male, just like the relationship between keys and keyholes. What would have caused him to make this demonstrable mistake? Is this not a paradigm case of the dependence of 'the real' upon 'the cultural'?

I think we need to combine this question arising from historical material with one that arises from cultural comparison. Why did ancient

Greeks and Chinese make sense of the body so differently? Here we have at least four different concepts of the body (i.e. those of the ancient Chinese, ancient Greeks, Renaissance anatomists and our own contemporaries). Can we say which of these is the truest? We might confidently respond that our contemporaries have the most effective, if not the most definitively true concept. I do not want to challenge this response. Here I only want to point out that the medical understandings of the four groups differ according to culturally and historically constructed concepts of the body.

Healing art as a system of practice

Depending on the kind of body concept that prevails in a specific society, a dominant style of healing art will also prevail. For example, where the body is thought to be composed of channels of ch'i (氣), healing art is to be directed toward adding or subtracting ch'i according to its guiding principles. Where the body is thought to be composed of four principal humours, the healing art is directed forward regaining harmony by bleeding, purging or vomiting. When we liken the body to a machine, the healing procedure is directed toward repairing the mechanical parts of the body machine.

However, in practice people do not depend solely on conceptually acceptable therapy. They tend not to care whether or not a certain therapy conforms to a particular conceptual structure, so long as it helps to improve their condition. In other words, people have had practical wisdom that does not necessarily depend upon theoretical reason. For example, the English sanitary revolution that was led by Chadwick in the 1840s is based not on a demonstrable theory of infection but on the ambiguous concept of miasma. Even so, it had a major impact on reducing infectious diseases as well as improving living conditions. The current increasing interest in alternative medicine provides another indicator which shows that in their behaviour people do not always strictly depend on scientifically verified therapies.

In other cases, people from different cultures or historical eras have used similar treatment methods for different theoretical reasons. Craniotomy (making a surgical opening in the skull) is probably one of the oldest surgical procedures that humans have ever performed. According to archaeologists, skulls with craniotomy scars are found throughout the world, ranging chronologically from the prehistoric era to the recent past. Were these dangerous operations being performed in order to reduce intracranial pressure caused by bleeding or tumours, as we do today? We do not know how they reached the conclusion that this operation needed to be performed. Nonetheless, we could speculate about this. Most historians of medicine believe that craniotomy was undertaken in order to expel an evil spirit that was thought to be residing in the brain. We could easily imagine that most patients would have died shortly after the operation, due to faulty diagnosis and primitive surgical skills. We do not know whether the diagnoses were right or wrong. However, according to archaeologists and archaeopathologists we can say for certain that some patients survived for quite a long time – long enough to show a healed bony margin after the operations. Moreover, the survival rate of craniotomised patients in the ancient and prehistoric era was much higher than that in medieval times.

In summary, we can make three points. First, people do not rely exclusively on theoretically acceptable methods when dealing with illnesses. They have practical wisdom as well as theoretical reason, and experience is as important as knowledge. Secondly, different systems of healing can propose exactly the same treatment method while providing completely different explanations. Thirdly, perhaps we would not be wholly justified in believing that our ancestors had a substantially inferior system of healing practice compared with our contemporaries.

Healing art as a personified virtue

Medical ethics was never a separate discipline from medicine until recently. It has always been a part of the healing art. We have the Hippocratic Oath in the West and Sun Simio's (孫思邈) code of ethics in the East, both originating thousands of years ago, and they were integral parts of the entire healing art, rather than being a separate subject of investigation. In East Asian tradition, the healing art has been the embodiment of Tao – that is, the sum total of good understanding, considerate and humane practice and virtue emanating from the person of the healer. These three are so tightly interconnected that none of them can be separated from the others. Humane practice is impossible without good understanding and good will on the part of the healer. The virtue of the healer cannot be cultivated without good understanding and experience derived from practice. One could argue that the situation has been the same in the West – that the separation of science from art, and of theory from practice, has been a relatively recent phenomenon. The Greeks also had the concept of embodied knowledge, if not exactly that of Tao. However, the ways in which these values were embodied were not entirely the same.

Let me explain this by citing two representative morality tales from the East and the West. The representative story demonstrating the basic attitude toward morality in the East is that of a thief who broke into a house to steal valuables. He saw a little boy playing in the back yard, and the child was about to fall into a well. What did the thief do? He completely forgot what had brought him there, and he saved the child. This is the compassionate mindset that everyone is believed to have, and it has become one of the main principles of Confucian morality.

The representative morality tale from the West is that of a Good Samaritan. Although the Samaritan was only a passer-by and a despised outsider, immediately upon finding a robbed and wounded stranger, he not only saved the man's life but also helped him to find food and shelter. This story has become the paradigm of Christian ethics.

What are the differences between the two representative stories? First, while Confucians assume that even a thief *inherently* has good will to save a child, Christians seem to assume that good will is to be praised and cultivated, but is not inherent. Secondly, the heroes of the two stories have quite different backgrounds. The hero of the East is a poor and blameworthy thief, while the hero of the West is a rather wealthy but despised merchant. We can say that the morality of Confucianism is a revelation of inherent virtues which everyone (even a thief) holds within themselves, while Christian morality comes from renewed consciousness that we (even Samaritans) are all neighbours. These contrasting features may have effects that last well into the present. And now both the East and the West are in need of each other's moral prototype.

East and West, then and now

Our journey from East to West and from past to present has nearly come to an end. Now it is time for us to reflect upon ourselves. What have we gained from this journey? In order to answer this question, we must first know in what context we are situated. We are at the beginning of the twenty-first century. And we have had an epochal announcement that the draft map of the human genome – God's secret code, as it were – has been completed. In conjunction with information technology, biotechnology is generally accepted as the key element for the future. Scientists have already cloned mammals, and it is said that cloning humans is a problem not of technique but of ethics. Accordingly, the concept of the human body is about to change from a structurally predetermined entity to a flexible and malleable form of life. In this scheme, a healing art is nothing more than a technique for repairing faulty parts of genes. Why then take the trouble to look around at the outdated healing arts of East and West? There seems to be no need to resort to the past or to an Eastern way of thinking, because the healing art has now become a laboratory procedure.

However, this conclusion would be unwarranted, chiefly because modern genetics is based on assumptions that seem to be heavily charged with cultural bias. One of these cultural assumptions is the habitual dichotomy between form and matter, which is evident neither in the West of the past nor in the East in general. This separation of essence from the messy sundries of phenomena has been the driving force behind scientific development, and it has been a great success. Biomedicine's success story was so powerful that people wanted to extrapolate the recent success story to the future. The optimistic perspective of biomedicine proposes a cultural milieu which considers the healing art to be merely repair work. However, this extrapolation is not justifiable either scientifically or philosophically. (We cannot discuss this point further here, although I guess that this will be an important topic in the history of biomedicine.) We are in a conceptual quandary in the midst of optimistic fervour. I hope that any insight we might have gained from our journey will help us to cope with that quandary and to come up with novel ideas for the future.

Remember that the purpose of our journey was to turn our assumptions upside down. We did this by re-evaluating what we are accustomed to, from a viewpoint that has been alien to us. By doing so we would be able to find out what is specific to biomedicine, rather than what was wrong in ancient or Eastern healing arts. Finally, let us ask a question that seems odd from the present common-sense view. What kind of assumptions does biomedicine have? Is it really culture free? In trying to answer these questions we could raise yet another one. Instead of asking whether or not the healing art of a specific era is *scientifically true*, we need to ask how well the healing art of an era is incorporated with the general culture of that era.

References

Kleinman AM (1993) What is specific to Western medicine? In: WF Bynum and R Porter (eds) *Companion Encyclopedia of the History of Medicine. Volume 1*. Routledge, London.

Lupton D (1996) *Medicine as Culture: illness, disease and the body in Western societies*. Sage, London.

Unschuld PU (1985) *Medicine in China: a history of ideas*. University of California Press, Berkeley, CA.

The registrar walked back into Accident and Emergency and asked a nurse to supplement the dressing on his thumb.

'I think we'd better just change the whole thing,' said the nurse, motioning to the doctor to follow him into the nearest cubicle. 'That's bleeding pretty freely. Do you think you could apply some pressure yourself here, while I get some more dressing on the wound?'

The nurse removed the dressing, cleaned away the blood, and formed a neat bandage around the doctor's hand.

'Looks good, and feels right,' he said. 'Nice neat job. I'd like to be able to do it like that.'

'Thanks – glad you appreciate it,' smiled the nurse. 'I like to get the art as well as the science right, if I can.'

'The aesthetics of nursing, eh?'

'The aesthetics of nursing. And of clinical care in general. Even in A & E.'

What has Art got to do with it? The aesthetics of clinical practice

Paul Wainwright

Introduction

Many people, if asked what they understand about aesthetics, would say that it was concerned with the nature of beauty and, in particular, the study of fine arts (by which most people would probably mean painting, sculpture, music, architecture and perhaps drama, literature and one or two others). Certainly a quick browse in the philosophy section of the library would reinforce this assumption, with many books having titles that clearly relate to aesthetics and the fine arts. Aschenbrenner and Isenberg (1965), to take one at random, would be typical, with the title *Aesthetic Theories: studies in the philosophy of art.*

What, then, has aesthetics got to do with healthcare practice or the philosophy of medicine? A quick search for the term 'aesthetics' on Medline turns up several thousand references, but nearly all of them are concerned with cosmetic surgery, cosmetic dentistry or the cosmetic results of other types of surgery. This is clearly an important area. There is no need to explore contentious examples such as breast implants for glamour models or face lifts for ageing film stars to recognise the place of cosmetic surgery in mainstream healthcare. The correction of a hare lip and cleft palate or reconstructive surgery following disfiguring treatment for cancer would seem to have obvious benefits beyond mere vanity, and any patient undergoing an invasive procedure can expect the surgeon to take reasonable care to achieve the best cosmetic result possible when closing a surgical incision or repairing trauma.

However, the cosmetic results of surgery are perhaps of less relevance to the philosophy of medicine. There are two other areas (at least) that are potentially more interesting, and these are the ones I wish to explore in more detail. The first is the idea that our understanding of aesthetics may have something to tell us about the nature, and our experience of, *illness itself*. The second is the idea that *practice* – the work and the actions or behaviour of the healthcare professional as it might be observed by the patient or a third party – is also of aesthetic interest.

'art' and 'Art'

It is important to clarify one or two issues. The first of these is concerned with questions about the nature of healthcare practice and whether any of the various forms of practice (medicine, nursing, physiotherapy, and so on) might usefully be described as an art or a science. For example, many authors have referred to the art and science of medicine, but I am going to leave aside the question of whether medicine, nursing, midwifery or any other healthcare trade should be thought of as a science, rather than just as the application of science for a specific purpose. This is an interesting question and may well be worth pursuing, but I do not intend to address it here.

Are the various forms of healthcare practice 'arts', and does art in that sense have anything to do with aesthetics? My response to this question is that it depends on what you mean by 'an art'. It is worth remembering that the use of the word 'art' to denote the fine arts, art with a capital 'A', is a relatively recent phenomenon, dating from the eighteenth century. The Latin root *ars*, and the Greek *techne* pre-date this usage by a considerable period, but if we think of words like 'artefact', 'artisan', 'technique', 'technician' and so on, we can see the influence of this original usage. For the ancient civilisations an art was any activity that was capable of being performed more or less well, and that required technique, expertise, skill and judgement. Activities that were regarded as arts were those that could not be done by rote or reduced to patterns of thoughtless habit.

The Greek and Latin terms therefore do not denote fine art in the modern sense. They were applied to all kinds of human activities that are now called crafts or sciences. The ancients always understood 'art' to mean something that could be taught and learned. The Greeks contrasted 'art' with 'nature', thinking of human activity in general, comparing artefacts made by people with natural objects or events that occurred without human intervention. Plato put art above routine because an art proceeds by rational principles and rules, while Aristotle listed art among the intellectual virtues, as an activity based on knowledge. For the Stoics, an art was a system of cognition, and a moral virtue was an art of living.

Even up to the middle of the eighteenth century we can see this general use of the term 'art'. For example, the French philosopher Abbé Batteux says 'In general, an art is a collection or assemblage of rules for doing well what can be done well or badly, because what can only be done well or done badly has no need of art' (Batteux, 1997, p. 103). He goes on to describe three kinds of art. The mechanical arts meet 'the basic needs of mankind', and provide solutions to problems – solutions which could be developed and perfected for future use. The other two types of art are the fine arts, which produce pleasure, and the arts that are both useful and agreeable, such as architecture.

Another eighteenth-century writer, Jean le Rond D'Alembert (1997), makes a similar claim:

In general, the name Art may be given to any system of knowledge which can be reduced to positive and invariable rules independent of caprice or opinion. In this sense it would be permitted to say that several of our sciences are arts when they are viewed from their practical side.

(D'Alembert, 1997, p. 107)

He also distinguishes between the mechanical arts and the liberal arts. Among the liberal arts, those that *imitate* are the fine arts, as opposed to the more useful liberal arts, such as grammar, logic and ethics.

Thus medicine, nursing and other healthcare occupations are clearly arts in this sense of the word. They involve techniques, things that require skill, and they cannot be done by rote or habit, or at least, they cannot be done well in this way. However, they are not fine arts by any modern understanding of that phrase.

Aesthetics

I suggested earlier that philosophical aesthetics is often taken to be concerned with theories of art and our appreciation of beauty in the fine arts. If this were the case, aesthetics would have little relevance for everyday experience. However, anyone who has ever considered the beauty of a landscape or remarked on the ugliness of an industrial site has already considered the possibility of an aesthetic experience that goes beyond the gallery or the museum. Cazeaux (2000) claims that aesthetics:

… has undergone a radical transformation in the last hundred years. Traditionally the subject has always occupied the margins of philosophy, for the simple reason that it deals with those aspects of experience which are the least amenable to categorisation, i.e. art, beauty, emotion, and the ever-changing delights of the senses. However, the divisions imposed on reality by modern reason and changes brought about by the industrialisation of experience have necessitated a rethinking of the relationship between the individual and reality. Gone are the notions of a distinct self in receipt of a mind-independent world and, in their place, are theses to the effect that consciousness and reality are interconnected at a fundamental level. One consequence of this shift is that aesthetic experience is redefined. Far from being a mere adjunct to everyday perception, it is shown to be vital to an understanding of the relationship between mind and world. The aesthetic, formerly exiled from mainstream attention, assumes centre-stage as the region to which we can turn for new cognitive possibilities and a sensibility that is critical of the divisions exercised by modern thought.

(Cazeaux, 2000, p. xiii)

Cazeaux's argument is crucial to our understanding of the place of aesthetics in healthcare, particularly his claim that aesthetic experience is 'vital to an understanding of the relationship between mind and world'. However, his suggestion that aesthetics has undergone a radical transformation in the last 100 years seems ironic, because the idea of aesthetics as exiled from mainstream attention is itself a relatively recent one. Beauty was not understood in ancient thought in the same way as it is in modern times. Greek and Latin writers never neatly or consistently distinguished beauty from the moral good. Plato, in the *Symposium* and the *Phaedrus*, speaks not merely of the beauty of human individuals but also of beautiful habits of the soul and beautiful cognitions, but he does not mention works of art at all. When the Stoics connected beauty and goodness, Kristeller (1997) suggests that by beauty they meant nothing but moral goodness. Later, beauty began to assume aesthetic significance, but never in the modern sense.

Whether we can speak of aesthetics in the case of Plato, Plotinus or Augustine will depend on our definition of that term, but we should certainly realise that in the theory of beauty, a consideration of the arts is quite absent in Plato and secondary in Plotinus and Augustine.

(Kristeller, 1997, pp. 91–2)

More recently, John Dewey (1934) protested at the way in which aesthetic appreciation had been hijacked by the fine arts and divided off into a compartment that referred to a very narrow range of experience, and he argued strongly for the recognition of the aesthetic in everyday life. Many of Dewey's examples are concerned with human activity, and thus with artefacts. However, natural phenomena are also valued for their aesthetic qualities. A contemporary American philosopher, Paul Ziff, concludes that 'anything that can be viewed is a fit object for aesthetic attention' (Ziff, 1997, p. 29), adding his voice to the strong opposition to the idea that aesthetics is confined to the study of beauty and the fine arts.

This opposition is not surprising, given that aesthetics derives from the Greek for perception, and was typically used to refer to what is valuable about experiences as *perceptual* experiences. As human beings we are constantly exposed to sensory data – to what William James called the blooming, buzzing confusion of stimuli (James, 1902). However, as human beings we also seek to organise these stimuli into some kind of order. Philosophers differ in their explanations of this process, but broadly speaking, the stimuli that we receive are organised or intuited into particular objects, and these in turn are further organised into general concepts. This is not, I would suggest, a neutral activity. Arranging our perceptions into recognisable objects and labelling them is an active process – an imposition of an order – that is constructed by ourselves. Our ability to do it at all depends, of course, on our prior experience – for how could we interpret or understand anything presented to us, other than by reference to previous experiences? If, while pointing at the horizon, we draw attention to 'a sunset', we are applying a concept that depends upon human ideas and values, a human interpretation of the phenomena that we perceive when heavenly bodies follow their mechanical paths and, not least, our prior experience of what usually takes place in a certain part of the sky at a particular time of the day. This process of interpretation also involves value judgements. We select which stimuli to attend to and which to ignore, and which elements to include in our representation of an object. Moreover, we express satisfaction or dissatisfaction with the results.

Thus our perceptions of the world require knowledge and effort, and this effort is repaid. If we are confronted with a novel situation, we will seek to make sense of it by reference to previous experiences that might in some way be similar, but our understanding and the quality of our perceptual experience will in the future be different if we have taken the trouble to find out something about the situation in question. Even the situations that we encounter frequently will be experienced differently depending on how they are presented in the context of our education, social and cultural norms, previous satisfactory or unsatisfactory experiences, our mood on the day, and so on. And we bring our own attention, our own willingness to engage with the thing (or situation) – the effort that we put into organising the experience, interpreting it and evaluating it makes any object's aesthetic quality as much a characteristic of the observer as of the object itself. Ziff illustrates this with clever interplay between descriptions of an alligator and of a painting by Leonardo:

> Seen from the side, the gator appears to have a great healthy grin conveying a sense of well-being vitality. When Ginevra's portrait was painted by Leonardo she must have been sick for a long time. The pallor of her face conveys a 'sense of melancholy'. The ossified scutes along his back forming the characteristic dermal armour constitute a powerful curving reticular pattern conveying simultaneously an impression of graceful fluidity and of remorseless solidity. Ginevra's face is 'framed by cascading curls. These ringlets, infinitely varied in their shapes and movement, remind us of Leonardo's drawings of whirling eddies of water'. He has just come out of the water to bask in the sun. His sight is acute, as is his power of hearing. But his eyes now have a lazy look, being half-closed, for he has upper and lower lids as well as a nictating membrane. Ginevra too stares at us out of half-closed eyes. He is not strabismic. Her eyes are hazel. His seem green and remote, despite the great grin.
>
> (Ziff, 1984, cited in Feagin and Maynard, 1997, p. 29)

To take stock of the argument so far, if we accept that the term 'aesthetic' is used to refer to what is *valuable* about *perceptual* experiences, we have to agree with Ziff that anything that can be viewed – anything of which we have a perceptual experience – can be capable of triggering an aesthetic response. There seems to be no good reason to deny this, and there are no criteria by which to segregate those perceptual experiences that I might consciously judge for their value from those that I might not consciously evaluate. Indeed, it is difficult to imagine a perceptual experience that *could not* be judged for its value in this way.

Aesthetics and the representation of illness

It may at first seem odd to talk about disease and illness in terms of an aesthetic appreciation. After all, disease is typically thought of as bad, unpleasant, ugly and undesirable. However, if we accept the richer view of aesthetics – that it is about far more than just the appreciation of works of art – and if we realise, as obviously we must, that any value judgement which has beauty at one end of the scale must have something disagreeable at the other, the idea becomes less far-fetched. To judge something ugly is, after all, to evaluate it – albeit negatively.

If we then go further, and realise that in viewing illness or disease as an object of perception we are in effect engaging in a creative act – producing a representation, unique on that occasion, which consists of selected elements brought together in the mind – then we can begin to see the relationship between aesthetics and our intuitions. If we agree that it is not only art objects that are fit for aesthetic attention, but also (as Ziff claims) anything that can be *viewed* and considered, and if we agree that diseases or illnesses can be viewed or considered, then diseases and illnesses must be fit for aesthetic attention. Of course, value judgements that an object is agreeable or disagreeable, beautiful or ugly, are just that – value judgements. The bee visiting the flower, as far as we can tell, makes no such judgement. The white clover infiltrating the lawn may delight or infuriate human observers or leave them unmoved, depending on their point of view, but to the bee the clover is merely a source of nectar. Judgements that flowers are beautiful, or that weeds spoil a lawn are necessarily human evaluations – expressions of human preferences for one thing over another. Aesthetic appreciation is, as far as we know, a distinctively human characteristic.

The discussion so far has referred to disease and illness as if they were independent entities that we can observe in some detached way. However, the aesthetic relationship is rather more complex than this. Byron Good argues that, in conventional terms of aesthetics:

> The aesthetic object is not reducible to the oil on the canvas or to a musical score or even its performance. It is also not reducible to a representation or reflection of these in the mind of the viewer or the musical audience. The aesthetic object is a particularly complex and dynamic form of relationship among these, a relationship which depends upon and yet transcends both performance and audience, reader and text, material object and a reflective, sensuous response.
>
> (Good, 1994, p. 167)

Good suggests, by analogy, that disease is not simply a state of the body, and neither is it just a reflection of that state in the experience of the sufferer or in the medical literature. Disease, according to Good's account, is 'a complex and dynamic form of relationship' between the experience of the patient, the literature, the conversations and opinions of doctors, the information produced by technologies, the opinions of the social world, and the views expressed through administrative and policy documents, tables of classification of diseases, and so on. Disease is thus 'a synthetic object *par excellence*'.

Why is this important? Drawing from literary theory, Good compares our perception of disease with the reading of a novel. If we follow a story, we do not simply receive the facts as they are set down. According to reading response theory, Good points out, we compose the story ourselves as we read. We create the plot as we proceed through a text, and through a form of aesthetic synthesis the story comes into being. According to this view there are two aspects of plot, namely the underlying structure of the story and the activity of the reader who imaginatively makes sense of the story. Characters in stories are not natural objects – they require the 'synthesising activities of readers' for their emergence. For Good, illness can be understood as narrative, and like the character in the plot 'it can never be ... comprehended in a single moment or from a single point of view' (Good, 1994, p. 167).

As with plots, narratives and characters, no two experiences of a disease will ever be precisely the same. Thus any account of illness and disease has somehow to deal with the complexity of illness as experienced by those involved – continually created through an aesthetic synthesis, always changing and unfolding, and never fixed.

Therefore the importance of an aesthetic response to illness and disease is that it necessarily involves value judgements about our perceptions and experiences. This stands in sharp contrast to the biomedical account of disease, which seeks to define it solely by reference to physiological measures, explicitly excluding any aspect of human preference or value judgement. Aesthetics gives us an alternative way of thinking about disease or illness, in which the necessarily human, *experiential*, side is not lost or downplayed.

The aesthetic appreciation of healthcare practice

If disease and illness demand an aesthetic appreciation, what can we say about the practice of healthcare practitioners? We may give a very similar account of practice to the one we have given of disease. Indeed, it would appear that we have no option but to give an aesthetic response to our experience of practice, since it would seem difficult to imagine a perceptual experience that was value free. The question is, what is the status or importance of this aesthetic response? Is it merely a curious, accidental phenomenon (perhaps a distraction from the more serious judgements we might make about practice)? Or is it central to our understanding of practice and, in particular, of what we might call good practice? Just as our understanding of illness is constituted through a variety of perspectives, so also practice will be viewed and synthesised from many perspectives. The recipient of care will have one view, the practitioner will have another, a third-party observer will have yet another, and the politicians, policy makers and managers will have different views again. In every case, the vision of practice will be generated from different sets of elements, from different values and perspectives, and from different knowledge bases.

When we observe the practice of a healthcare professional we tend to do so critically and to make some evaluation of it – as good or bad, the kind of practice to which we would like to be exposed or which we would prefer to avoid. We generally have some appreciation of it, and this appreciation tends to form along certain dimensions. For example, we may marvel at the skill, expertise and erudition of the practitioner. The diagnostic skills of the practitioner, piecing together the elements of the diagnostic puzzle, can be as impressive as any detective novel. The doctor inserts the lumbar puncture needle, the surgical nurse performs complex dressing techniques, the theatre nurse manages the instrument set and the swab count, the physiotherapist working in the stroke unit helps a patient return to independence, the palliative care specialist judges just the right combination of drugs to control the patient's symptoms, and the general practitioner listens to the patient and divines the nature of her problem.

We may also make an ethical assessment, recognising the difficulty of making decisions about the continuation or withdrawal of life-saving treatment – admiring the courage and honesty, the care and compassion, and the sense of justice displayed by doctors, nurses and other therapists. However, a full account of an episode of healthcare practice would seem to be incomplete if it described only the technical skills and the ethical conduct of the practitioner. When we come away from an episode of care and think about it, we might want to say something about how much we admired what the practitioner did, how observing that care made us feel, and how we responded to it at an emotional level. Here we are making an aesthetic judgement. After all, to admire something is to marvel at it appreciatively, with esteem or in the most vivid cases even with wonder or reverence. If observing a healthcare practice rouses in us such a sense of wonder or esteem, and induces in us an emotional response, then does that not sound very like an aesthetic contemplation? Thus there is something about our observation of healthcare practice that is concerned with our perceptual experience, and with the way in which we create and value that experience.

I mentioned John Dewey earlier, in the context of the more general understanding of aesthetics in everyday life. Dewey distinguishes between 'experience' and '*an* experience', the former being continuous but inchoate, whereas *an* experience occurs when what is experienced 'runs its course to fulfilment'.

A piece of work is finished in a way that is satisfactory; a problem receives its solution; a game is played through; a situation, whether that of eating a meal, playing a game of chess, carrying on a conversation, writing a book, or taking part in a political campaign, is so rounded out that its close is a consummation and not a cessation. Such an experience is a whole and carries with it its own individualising quality and self-sufficiency. It is *an* experience.

(Dewey, 1934, p. 47, original emphasis)

Dewey's claim is that the episodes that count as 'an experience' are the ones that are worthy of aesthetic appreciation. These are the ones to which we respond at an emotional level, and which we value and admire. He gives the example of watching a craftsman at work, noting the attention to what he is doing, the concentration, the commitment to doing the job well and producing something of worth and distinction.

This reminds us that the recognition of what counts as '*an* experience' requires work on the part of the observer. Whether I am watching the blacksmith in his forge or the surgeon in the operating theatre, I have to make sense of what I am seeing. From the 'blooming, buzzing mass of stimuli' I must determine which ones to attend to and how to draw them together in a representation. I intuit the situation, filtering out and ignoring what I take to be extraneous information, and constructing the experience for myself. I may, of course, be mistaken. Is that the kindly GP I see beside the patient in her chair, giving her an injection to relieve her symptoms, or is it the murderer Shipman? I may marvel at the achievements of the surgeon when others dismiss him as a clumsy butcher. I may recognise the skill with which the nurse develops a relationship of trust with a patient and transforms his attitude to his illness, setting him on a course of recovery and return to independence, but only because I am attuned to the subtle cues of expression, attention, body language and tone of voice. In forming these representations and making judgements about them I am influenced by my own knowledge and experience – not only of the direct clinical picture in front of me, but also potentially by every other aspect of my experience in life to date. Whether I perceive the doctor who is talking to the surgeon as a kindly physician with the patient's best interests at heart, or as an arrogant, paternalistic professional who is disregarding the patient's autonomy, exploiting the imbalance in the power relationship between the professions and the laity, will depend among other things on my political views, and possibly my age, sex, ethnic origin and the dominant culture in which I was brought up. It will also depend on the views of others who may be influential in forming opinions about professional practice. Inevitably, though, I will form some value judgement about my perception of what I have seen, and this will be an aesthetic judgement.

Conclusions and further questions

If we accept the foregoing account (of the reception of stimuli, the intuition of objects, the creation of the representation of the particular and its recognition as a member of a group of concepts, the creative work involved in this, and the evaluation of the quality of this perceptual experience) then we must be committed to the presence of the aesthetic in all aspects of our daily lives, and in particular in the context of this chapter, to the importance of the aesthetic in our understanding of illness and disease and of the practice of healthcare practitioners.

The presence of the aesthetic in our perceptions of healthcare may be inescapable, but is it important, or is it merely a curiosity, or even a nuisance – an unwanted intrusion into what should be a world of objectivity and science, a world that is usually at pains to exclude subjective elements of experience? Alternatively, could it even have therapeutic value? I would like to suggest that this may well be the case.

The problem for most of us is that much of the time we simply do not attend to the aesthetic dimension of our experiences, and indeed we filter out or selectively ignore much of the world that is available to us to experience. There are probably many good psychological reasons for this. However, if we are involved in healthcare we have a responsibility to be sensitive to the quality of the service that we deliver, and this must mean that we have an obligation to be aware of and to respond to the aesthetic quality of practice, as well as our aesthetic response to the experience of illness and disease.

It seems entirely reasonable to suggest that, for example, the kind of 'experience' that Dewey describes would also be exemplified by the experience of watching the skilled practitioner at work. The general practitioner who is taking infinite pains to be clear about what is really troubling the patient and to find ways to offer help, the nurse who is making the critically ill patient comfortable, or the surgeon who is performing a technically difficult procedure calmly and confidently, might all give us the same aesthetic response as Dewey's blacksmith. And if the qualities that are encapsulated in these (admittedly caricatured) vignettes capture what we might call 'good practice', then their aesthetic quality provides us with an important criterion by which to judge the quality of care.

It also seems reasonable that, from the recipient's point of view, care that gives aesthetic satisfaction may have other benefits. If being cared for in this way makes one feel good, and gives one the impression that one is important and considered worthy of such attention, who knows what benefits may follow (e.g. for the immune system). Mercer *et al.* (2001), in a study in the outpatient department of a homeopathic hospital, found that the extent to which patients felt 'enabled' by their consultation was significantly correlated with their perception of the doctor's level of empathy. It has been suggested that, among cancer patients with an uncertain prognosis, those patients who are popular with the nurses may have better rates of survival than those who are not (Goldie, 1990). There is other, anecdotal, evidence that women with breast cancer who attend relaxation classes have a better survival rate that those who do not. The patient who feels liked, cared for, or even loved may, like the patient who is able to enter a state of deep relaxation, find strength on which to draw, while the patient who feels unpopular and uncared for may not only lack access to this source of strength, but may actually feel undermined.

It certainly seems to be the case that patients have the ability to differentiate between those professionals whom they perceive to be more caring and those whom they perceive to be less so (Brown, 1986). Both the way in which professionals construct their relationships with patients, and the way in which patients construct their relationships with their illness and with their carers, inevitably involve the aesthetic – in ways that we do not fully understand.

References

Aschenbrenner K and Isenberg A (1965) *Aesthetic Theories: studies in the philosophy of art*. Prentice-Hall, London.

Batteux A (1997) The fine arts reduced to a single principle. In: S Feagin and P Maynard (eds) *Aesthetics*. Oxford University Press, Oxford.

Brown L (1986) The experience of care: patient perspectives. *Topics Clin Nurs*. **8**: 56–62.

Cazeaux C (2000) *The Continental Aesthetics Reader*. Routledge, London.

D'Alembert J le R (1997) The arts and the fine arts. In: S Feagin and P Maynard (eds) *Aesthetics*. Oxford University Press, Oxford.

Dewey J (1934) *Art as Experience*. Pedigree, New York.

Feagin S and Maynard P (eds) (1997) *Aesthetics*. Oxford University Press, Oxford.

Goldie L (1990) Ethical dilemmas for nurses and their emotional implications. In: *APP Conference Proceedings*. The Association for Psychoanalytic Psychotherapy in the NHS, London.

Good B (1994) *Medicine, Rationality and Experience: an anthropological perspective*. Cambridge University Press, Cambridge.

James W (1902) The principles of psychology; http://psychclassics.yorku.ca/James/Principles/prin13.htm

Kristeller PO (1997) The modern system of the arts. In: S Feagin and P Maynard (eds) *Aesthetics*. Oxford University Press, Oxford.

Mercer S, Reilly D and Watt G (2001) *Enablement and the Therapeutic Alliance: an evaluation of the consultation at the Glasgow Homeopathic Hospital.* ADHOM, Glasgow.

Ziff P (1997) Anything viewed. In: S Feagin and P Maynard (eds) *Aesthetics.* Oxford University Press, Oxford.

'Well, that was a clean dressing three minutes ago – but it certainly isn't now. Look, I think you've cut into an artery. Someone needs to take another look at this.'

The nurse left the room to call the duty consultant. After a while an elderly-looking doctor came in and greeted the registrar. She looked at the thumb carefully.

'I'm going to open it up a bit more and tie off that artery,' she said. 'How much movement do you have in the thumb? ... Good, it's basically OK. Though I'd definitely want to see it later – do get it checked, won't you – once the wound has healed up.'

The nurse prepared the doctor's hand and the consultant began to explore the wound.

'Well, the artery has indeed been cut; but don't worry, young man – we'll sort it right away. I think it will be right as rain in about ten days or so. We can never be entirely confident, of course', she went on. 'Human beings are so variable. Even when medically qualified. Well, I expect you can keep an eye on yourself, can't you?'

The consultant left, and the young doctor lay back on the couch wondering when – and if – he would regain full use of his thumb.

Do we really have to live with this?
Uncertainty in medicine

John Saunders

Life is short, the Art is long, Opportunity fleeting, Experiment dangerous and Judgement difficult.

(Hippocrates, *Aphorisms*, trad.)

Introduction

Doubt and uncertainty are daily elements of a doctor's work. If uncertainty really was all-pervasive, the result would paralyse all action – the doctor would never know what to do, and would therefore do nothing. Of course, doctors actually do a lot. Uncertainty does not paralyse – indeed it sometimes seems to inhibit certain doctors less than we might think desirable. Doctors have to cope with uncertainty, and it is a recognised part of their role to do so.

Consider the following examples.

Patient A has chest pain. It is described as severe and constricting, and the patient feels breathless. There is only a past history of an anxiety state. Nothing is found on examination and the patient does not appear to be in pain. An ECG is normal. The doctor is uncertain what the patient means by pain. Is this the anguish of cardiac ischaemia or is it the manifestation of hyperventilation syndrome with anxiety and panic? The doctor is not sure what the patient means.

Patient B has chest pain. It is severe and constricting, and the patient feels breathless. Perhaps there is the same past history but this time the patient appears to be in pain, sweaty and breathless. The ECG gives rise to suspicion of ischaemic change. This time the doctor is uncertain what to do because she does not know the agreed indications for clot-dissolving therapy (thrombolysis) in cardiac ischaemia. The doctor is uncertain because she does not know what is well known.

Patient C has chest pain. It is severe and constricting, and the patient feels breathless. This patient does have cardiac ischaemia and has received thrombolytic therapy. However, the pain recurs. The doctor is uncertain whether to transfer the patient to a tertiary centre 56 miles away for consideration of invasive treatment involving angioplasty (i.e. a balloon to distend the blocked artery and open it up). What might be best for this patient at such a distance? The doctor is uncertain what to do because no one knows. Clinical trials might show that such a treatment is valuable, but does the evidence of the trials apply to this patient in this place at this distance from a tertiary centre?

Patient D has chest pain. It is severe and constricting, and the patient feels breathless. This patient is also having a coronary thrombosis, like patient C, but he also has very advanced cancer. He is too distressed for rational discussion, even after pain relief. Previously the patient, who is now 88 years of age, said that he did not want heroic treatments and he hoped that he would soon die peacefully. The doctor is uncertain what to do, and whether it is right simply to give pain relief only or to institute a more active course of therapy. He knows what these therapies do, but he does not know which one would be appropriate for this patient.

These four examples demonstrate four different types of uncertainty. As a simple classification we might suggest the following.

1 Uncertainty in communication, or *interpersonal uncertainty:* Medicine is practised on people, and people have their own modes of expression, even when they share the same first language. Patient A, her doctor and her fellow patients may use language differently, they may exaggerate or downplay aspects of their stories, and their non-verbal communication may confirm or appear to deny what they are saying. They may not say what they mean. We might call this uncertainty in communication interpersonal uncertainty.

2 Lack of knowledge, or *uncertainty arising from ignorance:* Patient B's doctor in this example was simply ignorant. She did not know what she needed to know. Medicine is a vast and ever expanding body of knowledge. No one could possibly know everything that may be needed in a particular situation. However, there is no mystery about the uncer-

tainty here. The doctor needs to ask a colleague who is better informed, or consult a textbook. Uncertainty may result from ignorance, but at least in principle the answer is simple enough.

3 *Uncertainty in application:* Medicine is an applied science, and knowledge about the processes of disease or therapy must be applied to individuals. The evidence from the scientific literature may be excellent, but there may still be doubt as to whether it applies to the particular patient (in this case, patient C). We might give this the rather grand title of epistemological uncertainty (epistemology is the branch of philosophy concerned with knowledge). What might enable us to be certain about what is known for this patient? For example, would further studies of patients with this condition remove or reduce our uncertainty?

4 *Moral uncertainty:* If medicine is applied science, then a decision has to be made not just that it would be effective in a given situation but whether it would be effective in achieving a particular goal. What should be our goal in treating a particular patient and how could we determine it with confidence? Furthermore, who determines that goal? How can we be certain about this? For patient D, the goal might be treatment of the heart attack, but it might equally be a comfortable death. Let us call this moral (or ethical) uncertainty.

Interpersonal uncertainty

Interpersonal uncertainty arises from the lack of confidence we have in what has been said or what has been meant. We tend to assume that when a patient speaks to us, they tell us what their main concerns are. Frequently this simply is not true. The patient may be asked a series of closed questions that avoid the main problem, or they may not answer our question at all. If they are asked an open question, such as 'tell me about your concerns', the patient may recite a long tale of what a previous doctor has told them. All of this presents the skilled clinician with a challenge to draw out the information that is needed. In principle this is a task that can be taught and learned. Given that most diagnosis depends on history taking, it is hardly surprising that communications modules and courses have burgeoned in reformed medical curricula.

There are further subtle issues when the patient and the doctor come from significantly different cultural backgrounds (Dosani, 2003). Here gestures may carry different meanings. For example, the culture of an orthodox Jew may forbid him from shaking hands with a female doctor, in case she is menstruating. Words may be used in ignorance of their ambiguities – a simple example might be the description of a patient as 'not alcoholic', meaning that they do not drink alcohol, not that they have no alcohol problem. Effective understanding may sometimes demand a deep cultural understanding which may go beyond the words spoken to their context. Languages have subtle differences of meaning, and no one language can be completely translated into another. Even a patient or professional who is fluent in a second language may use modes of thought that are based on their first language.

Part of the benefit to the patient of a long association with a particular doctor, especially in the context of a chronic disease, is that the doctor and the patient know each other. This means that the significance for the patient of a particular complication or symptom can be rapidly put into the context of a life plan and its values, as these are known with some confidence by the professional. By contrast, if such a patient with a long-term problem is unknown to the doctor, the situation is charged with uncertainty. It is difficult to advise about anything – even if the consequences of that advice are known with certainty – if the doctor does not really know the patient.

And if we know what we mean by 'knowing' the patient, we mean much more than a set of propositions about them. Rather we are referring to a pattern of behavioural predictions, values, responses and so on. Some of this we can articulate, but much cannot be described verbally, most obviously physiognomy itself. We could not describe most of the people we know explicitly, yet we could pick them out from a crowd of hundreds of thousands. A close knowledge of someone will mean that we can pick out their responses by a knowledge of their character that will always go beyond the explicit. Our knowledge of them as individuals is at least partly tacit – that is, we cannot fully describe or explain what we in fact know.

Think of the task of drawing a face on the basis of a verbal description – it would not remotely resemble the person whom we had in mind when we offered the description to the artist. In the case of individuals, our knowledge of them comes as much from a constructive empathy and *indwelling* as from the explicit 'facts' of their behaviour, appearance or words – where 'indwelling' means the ability to put oneself in another's place, an act of imaginative sympathy. Our knowledge is necessarily always going to be incomplete – so great are the complexities of personality. Uncertainty is inevitable. For the doctor in an inner-city practice where each year 20% of patients may be replaced by other patients, uncertainty of an interpersonal kind will be a major problem in daily work – simply knowing the patient will be less likely.

We need to recall that our minds have no lexical reserves – no really specific or adequate vocabulary – to deal with extremes of human experience either in ourselves or in others. In the silence, cliché and jargon find their place, and we frequently resort to metaphor. The chest pain is 'a weight on the chest' or 'a knife stabbing' or 'a tiger tearing my chest apart' – regardless of the fact that those who have actually had a knife in the chest experience something rather different, and few have lived to describe the 'tiger'. Metaphor is central to description, and description is central to any full understanding of human experience, but especially pain and death. Metaphor may also offer the means of making sense of the experience. This may be especially true in terminal care, where it may be the means of assisting in the treatment and of having some control in a situation where control of other areas is diminishing inexorably. It may be the means of involving families and friends in the experience – of giving them the direction, the map of dying. TS Eliot wrote that 'The communication of the dead is tongued with fire beyond the language of the living.' Eliot is telling us that this experience goes beyond what our ordinary language can tell us.

Uncertainty arising from ignorance

Uncertainty resulting from ignorance is simple to resolve in principle – ask someone or look it up in a book or on the Internet – but of course the first step is to recognise such ignorance. Explicit scientific knowledge can usually be expressed in a series of propositions. Thus a few sentences ('propositions') can define what we mean by 'myocardial infarction', its treatment, its implications, and so on.

Such propositional knowledge cannot be stated without a *personal* component. If we say that 'the treatment for acute myocardial infarction starting less than 24 hours ago is thrombolysis', we are claiming that *we ourselves know* this. It is the nature of an assertion that it carries an emotional or personal commitment of this kind. For example, a doctor who is giving a serious diagnosis will feel the weight of a heavy personal responsibility – the more so according to the uncertainty of the information that he is about to transmit. A diagnosis of terminal cancer may be based on no more than the clinical presentation and examination. On the other hand, it may be based both on a typical clinical picture and on investigations such as X-rays, biochemical tests and biopsies. The weightier responsibility is upon the doctor who lacks the more detailed information.

When the information is serious, as with a terminal diagnosis, uncertainty may be felt even when the facts of the situation allow no other explanation. A patient may present with a fairly typical picture of malignant disease, perhaps with weight loss, enlarged lymph glands, an abnormal chest X-ray, and so on, yet most doctors still want a tissue sample – something seen under the microscope – to remove the last doubt, to be absolutely sure. Uncertainty is not an objective value. It is not something that we can measure, but a psychological state. If much hangs on the outcome, we want the evidence to be as watertight as possible. We want our patient's clinical picture to resemble that in the textbook as closely as possible.

Uncertainty in application

In our third type of uncertainty, the doctor thinks that he knows the facts of the situation. He knows the diagnosis with confidence, how far the disease has progressed, the patient's values and the scientific literature with its published data on investigation and treatment for that disease. However, even armed with a knowledge of such detailed facts, he is uncertain how to apply them. He may have an intimate knowledge of the established scientific laws that apply to a given clinical situation, but be uncertain what might be true for this paticular patient. Evidence has been graded as shown in Box 1.

Box 1

Level   Type of evidence

Ia   Evidence from a meta-analysis of randomised controlled trials

Ib   Evidence from at least one randomised controlled trial

IIa   Evidence from at least one well-designed controlled study without randomisation

IIb   Evidence from at least one other type of well-designed quasi-experimental study

III   Evidence from well-designed non-experimental descriptive studies, such as comparative studies, correlation studies and case-control studies

IV   Evidence from expert committee reports or opinions and /or clinical experiences of respected authorities

Source: US Agency for Health Care Policy and Research (1992).

However, even the evidence that comes from randomised controlled clinical trials may be of uncertain value in a given situation. For example, it has been shown that lowering blood pressure reduces the risk of stroke. It is also known that preventive measures are more likely to be of value when the risk is highest. Thus in theory we might think that a 90-year-old patient who will be at high risk is best treated for raised blood pressure. Unfortunately, there have been no randomised controlled trials of patients of this age. We can only extrapolate the known scientific facts from a younger group of patients.

Broadly speaking, we can classify clinical trials into two groups. In the *explanatory* or *exclusive design*, a simple law is being established. For example, does drug X lower blood pressure? In order to demonstrate this, a group of patients is selected that is as homogeneous as possible. Thus comorbidities are excluded, the age range is small, the gender is male only, ethnic minority groups are excluded, and so on. With a relatively small number of subjects, we can establish the effect of the drug on blood pressure easily and within a fairly short period of time. But how useful is this information? How far can the conclusions be extrapolated to the general population, or to those who are older or female or from ethnic minorities, etc.? We cannot be certain about this – we cannot *deduce* a conclusion from a proposition that is based on the selected population that participates in the study or trial to the individual patient. Rather, we may have to proceed using our common sense, whatever the power of the evidence. Our action may be reasonable, and in that sense rational, but it is not logically necessitated by the (more or less) certain evidence. In that sense, our action may be sensible or reasonable, but it is non-rational.

In the *pragmatic* or *inclusive design*, we may seek to include everyone who has the condition, regardless of comorbidities, age, gender, ethnicity and so on. This design may be attractive because it shows that the agent is effective in everyone, but in fact we face a similar problem of uncertainty. Does the successful outcome of the study apply to all of the groups of people in the trial, or have certain groups made a relatively larger contribution? Perhaps some subgroups do not benefit at all. However, even if this were shown to be the case in a particular study we would not have thereby explained the difficulty of extrapolation – we would simply have introduced a further problem. The problem of extrapolation persists even if all subgroups benefit equally, since clinical application must sooner or later concern patients who were not tested in the study itself. Thus the problem of extrapolation is incorrigible – the facts upon which clinical practice is based concern groups of people, and there can be no certainty, even in theory, of their applying to the individual in front of me. To that degree, uncertainty is not a regrettable psychological fact of life, but a necessary truth about the way things are – unalterably. It is the doctor's task then to commit himself to a belief in what is the case for this patient – a statement made responsibly and, based on his understanding of the evidence as far as it goes, with *universal intent*, which implies the conviction that although the evidence may be inadequate, another individual should reach the same conclusion in the same set of circumstances. In other words, the doctor believes his judgement to be *true*.

The shortcoming of the randomised trial is that its experimental design requires the recruitment of a group of volunteers who may not be typical of the type of patients who most commonly present with the problem under study. The trial studies a disease or its therapy removed from its context. One way to get round this problem is to conduct observational studies (Benson, 2000; Concato, 2000; Pocock, 2000). There is a continuing debate as to whether such studies produce similar results to those from randomised trials. Of course, their weakness is that the design is not experimental – each patient's treatment is chosen rather than randomly assigned, so there is an unavoidable risk of selection bias and of systematic differences in outcomes that are not due to the treatment itself. There is no way to be certain of the truth here. Both observational studies and trials may also suffer from recruitment quirks or problems with the delivery of treatment that cast doubt on the conclusions, and studies with negative findings may not be published at all (so-called *publication bias*). Uncertainty is something we cannot avoid, because we have no way of knowing what is true. As Plato expressed it (in the mouth of Meno):

> But how will you look for something when you don't in the least know what it is? How on earth are you going to set up something you don't know as the object of your search? To put it another way, even if you come right up against it, how will you know that what you have found is the thing you didn't know?
>
> Plato, *The Meno* (Guthrie, 1956, p. 128)

There is an alternative approach, namely the use of guidelines or protocols. These consist of consensus opinions on how to manage certain clinical situations or conditions, and are seen as a way to bring order into the chaos of widespread variations in diagnosis or treatment. Unfortunately, guidelines may represent no more than an attempt to impose a spurious rationality on an inherently irrational process. For example, diagnosis depends critically on the health beliefs and illness behaviour of the patient and the quality of the doctor–patient relationship. Diagnosis is also subject to bias because of availability error, in which the probability of a diagnosis seems to be higher if a doctor has just seen a series of patients with a particular disease and then sees another one with similar symptoms, or when a patient who knows someone with a set of symptoms of a particular serious disease is concerned that he or she may have it, too. What guidelines do offer is the reassurance that, despite uncertainty, a significant body of professional opinion will support the practitioner. This makes coping with uncertainty easier. Yet the good doctor will use guidelines as just that, and be willing to violate the guidance in particular cases if the circumstances are judged to differ in some significant way from those implied or stated in the guidelines.

Perhaps we know more than we can tell. In particular cases we may ignore items of the history, features of the examination or request particular investigations without being able to say explicitly why – and we were right to do so. However, we also realise that the more we discover, the more our ignorance confronts us. In Isaac Newton's phrase, 'I seem to have been only like a boy playing on the seashore and diverting myself in now and then finding a smoother pebble or a prettier shell than ordinary, whilst the great ocean of truth lay all undiscovered before me.' In clinical practice, even very basic things may be uncertain, and some that appear to be certain may seem to change. After 200 years the established place of digoxin in therapeutics has been challenged, and the debate has now continued for 30 years. We have further difficulties in devising a strategy of treatment for a patient when a multiplicity of treatments may have been validated, yet it is not clear when to use them. For example, thiazolidinedione drugs in diabetes may be best used early in the disease, but so might biguanides, and both types of drug may be used with other agents. Five different groups of drugs are available, so in theory we need outcome trials on all 120 possible combinations. However, this sort of information is never going to be available. The studies required would take too long, the expense of mounting them would be too great, and by the time they were complete they would be rendered obsolete by new medications coming on to the market. Instead we must traverse what have been called the 'grey zones of clinical practice' using rules of thumb, experience, commitment or information gleaned from other modes of study (e.g. observational trials, experimental models, rational extrapolations from presumed pathophysiology, etc.).

There is no logical or scientific way of deciding between minimalism or an intervention that is based on inference and experience. The consensus of the guideline writers is not itself 'evidence'. At best it is the summary of practical wisdom. Clinical reasoning, with its reliance on experience, extrapolation and the critical application of the other *ad hoc* rules described above, must be applied if we are to traverse the 'grey zones of clinical practice'.

Eliciting patient preferences is especially important when there is doubt about the best course of action. However, this is difficult with long-term treatments, when a patient's preferences may change as time passes, but decisions are needed now. A reflective practitioner treating hypertension or diabetes can hardly fail to be aware of this problem in daily practice. In conditions such as these, the trade-offs between probable short-term harm or inconvenience and possible long-term benefits are individual, difficult to quantify, full of uncertainty, and likely to change with life's changing circumstances.

Medicine would be difficult to practise without those daily non-scientific rules of thumb that guide decisions, when the doctor must cope with uncertainty in a particular situation. 'Ockham's razor' tells us to go to the simplest unifying hypothesis when diagnosing the patient's disease. If a patient has weakness in the legs, unsteadiness of gait and double vision, then we try to explain it as the result of one disease process rather than three separate ones. Sutton's law (based on the bank robber who told the judge he robbed banks because that is where the money is) similarly tells us to opt for the commonest explanation. If we are unable to explain a phenomenon then, all other things being equal, we would perform those tests that are directed at the common causes of the problem before the tests that are directed at the rare ones. Or we would look in those places that are presented to us – we might biopsy an enlarged liver, and not do tests on some other apparently normal part of the body. When we use extrapolation, we are employing a simple rule of thumb to cope with our uncertainties, and there is no logical necessity – no clear rule – with regard to the way we use this principle Practolol was shown to reduce deaths after acute myocardial infarction, but it was not until huge trials of other beta-blocking drugs had been conducted that the effect was accepted as one that could be extrapolated to other drugs in the group. By contrast, we have tended to assume that all effects of angiotensin-inhibitor drugs are a class effect, even if the specific licensing arrangements for drugs now discourage such assumptions as a guide to practice. We may not know the margins of benefit in a disease, so we tend to treat at an earlier stage, or we may believe that early treatment may have advantages despite the uncertainty of the subsequent development of the disease process. For example, gallstones may be removed even though it is uncertain that they are causing symptoms, on the grounds that they may cause problems in the future. Published evidence itself, however valuable, is not enough to resolve our uncertainties. All data, regardless of their completeness or accuracy, are interpreted by the clinician so that he or she can make sense of them and apply them in practice. Experts take into account 'messy' details, such as context, cost, convenience and the values of the patient. 'Doctor factors', such as emotions, bias, prejudice, risk aversion, tolerance of uncertainty and personal knowledge of the patient, all influence clinical judgement. It is impossible to make explicit all aspects of professional competence.

What of the evidence itself? What counts as evidence? The power of the randomised controlled trial is considerable, but even here judgements must be made that are not certain. Suppose that there is a trial of analgesics. What determines how we describe the pain that qualifies for the patient to enter the study? Would the outcome be different if a different criterion was used? Or in a surgical trial, how do we randomise for the experience and skill of the surgeon? Is it adequate to assume that after having performed a certain number of procedures, the level of skill will be the same? And how might this work in a cluster randomisation, when systematic bias can creep in even more easily? (In cluster randomisation, we may randomise according to a population rather than an individual – for example, we might randomise general practices to test the organisation of a particular screening method.) Who defines a pulmonary embolus, a myocardial infarct or schizophrenia, and why? Might the consensus be wrong? And how certain can it be? We could give many more examples. Certainty is not always possible – large, apparently well-designed trials have yielded results which are not universally accepted. For example, the Universities Group Diabetes Program was a large-scale trial of oral hypo-glycaemic agents in the treatment of diabetes involving several hundred patients, yet most believe that its conclusions were wrong, although it took over 20 years for them to be rebutted.

Living and working with uncertainty is uncomfortable. Often healthcare professionals do tests of little discriminating power because anything that might help, at however low a level of probability, seems better than proceeding with unaided judgement (e.g. brain scans for what are obviously tension headaches, heart monitoring for anxiety-related palpita-tions and so on). Alternatively, further opinions are requested, often invol-ving much time and expense. How uncertain does one have to be to order a repeat test, or to request a second, third or even fourth opinion? As public expectation rises, these behaviours that involve seeking greater certainty may be inevitable. Who decides what is reasonable in these circumstances? Should it be the taxpayer, the insurer, the professional or the patient? The search for epistemological certainty has a price. We have spent longer considering the uncertainty of application because of its importance in the daily lives of practising clinicians. In an age of 'evidence-based practice', it is of pressing importance to appreciate the limitations and uncertainties that cannot be resolved – even in principle – by 'evidence', however valuable that may be.

Moral uncertainty

Moral (or ethical) uncertainty typically occurs when we do not know what course of action to take for a patient, even though the possible courses of action are easy enough to define. For instance, this situation might arise because the patient is unable to express a preference due to incompetence, or because we are unsure how to present the facts to the patient – knowing that his or her preferences will be very largely determined by the way we describe the possibilities. If a treatment has a low chance of success, we may be unwilling to commend it with enthusiasm – not because we do not know the possibilities, but because we cannot bring to our recommendations the enthusiasm that is needed to convince the patient that this option might be worthwhile. Many would say that a 1% success rate for cardiopulmonary resuscitation hardly seems worthwhile, given that this procedure has a similar complication rate for causing a persistent vegetative state (which most would consider worse than death). Therefore we might attach words like 'pointless' or 'futile' to our description. Our uncertainty about what to do is coloured by our beliefs about the possible but uncertain, outcomes. It will be more uncertain whether an intervention should be offered to an unconscious patient. Should we feed an unconscious patient after a stroke? We do not know the patient's values, and there is no way of determining them. So what should we do? How can we cope with this uncertainty, knowing that by one course of action we may sentence the patient to a life that may have been considered by them to be worse than death, and by the other course of action we may sentence them to death itself? Such decisions involve overt value judgements, and where the professional attempts to determine the best interests of the incompetent patient, that judgement will always be uncertain.

The term 'judgement' carries a certain weight and seriousness. We might ask whether this is simply a way of supporting the uncertainties of belief as opposed to the certainties of knowledge. Knowledge is certain and cannot be false, whereas belief may well be uncertain or mistaken. This is not especially helpful. Knowledge may be certain and true for the same reason that 'treason never prospers'. We can say that treason never prospers, because if it does so then it is no longer called treason. If I was absolutely certain of something and then later on I concluded that it was false or even only doubtful, I would not now say that I knew it but was mistaken. Rather, I would say that I never really knew it at all. If 'I knew A', then I am implying first, that I was subjectively certain about A, secondly, that A is true, and thirdly, that I was objectively justified in being certain about A (Ewing, 1951). To assert that I knew A requires all three conditions to be fulfilled. For knowledge to be certain, we must be able to demonstrate that we may rely on it completely. Of course, there may still be cases of error which are *psychologically* indistinguishable from knowledge, and about which we are absolutely certain.

One further area of moral uncertainty deserves brief comment. This is the radical moral sceptic's view that there is no possibility of agreement about moral issues, even in principle, since the moral views of people in different cultures or societies are so different. According to such a view, all morality is uncertain and cannot be otherwise. There are three immediate responses to this. First, there is actually a considerable degree of moral consensus, as evidenced by such statements as the United Nations Universal Declaration of Human Rights. Secondly, no given human society could exist in harmony without some shared sense of morality. Thirdly, it makes no sense, logically speaking, to suppose that a particular view of morality is merely relative to a given society, while expecting all to subscribe to a general, absolute, non-relative requirement of respect, toleration or non-interference. In fact, we simply do not believe that eating or enslaving people, burning widows, gassing Jews, circumcising women, and so on, are somehow acceptable in certain societies while remaining unacceptable in our own. If uncertainties in morality or its basis are somehow more obvious to us than in science, that does not make our convictions any less important or worth acting on. Indeed, in daily medical practice we have little option but to act – because the patient is in front of us. Faced with the uncertainties of whether or not to withdraw the feeding tube, we do engage in discussion. We do not believe that this is merely an uncertain subjective judgement about which there is nothing more to be said. We would not be happy with a doctor who simply tossed a coin to determine his actions. Moral uncertainty may be common, but it is the nature of moral reflection to believe that there are right answers, otherwise morality as an enterprise would cease to exist.

Concluding remarks

Finally, then, uncertainty represents a problem for the patient (Ogden, 2002). One of the difficulties for patients in understanding what is proposed in clinical trials is uncertainty. Many patients really do believe that doctors know what to do in a given situation. Uncertainty under-mines the confidence that patients have in their doctors, and leads to outcomes that may be less desirable than when certainty is implied. Thus a group of 200 patients who presented in general practice with symptoms but no abnormal physical signs, and in whom no definite diagnosis was made, were randomly selected for one of four consultations (Thomas, 1987). In one group uncertainty was revealed, either with or without treatment, and no firm assurance was given: 'I cannot be certain what is the matter with you' or 'I am not sure that the treatment will have an effect.' In the other groups, a firm diagnosis was given and, where treat-ment was given, there was firm assurance of its effect. Nearly twice as many of those who received a positive consultation improved compared with those who were exposed to uncertainty. More recently, a study showed that expressions of uncertainty have a potentially detrimental effect on patients, and that patients and doctors have different ratings for the phrases that express uncertainty. Thus not only is uncertainty a daily reality of practice, but also we are uncertain even how to express it. If the content of communication is itself ethically difficult in the selection and ordering of (uncertain) facts, then so too is the language in which these facts are communicated. Nothing is certain except death and taxes, says the old saw (variously attributed). In medicine, the only certain practitioner or patient is the unthinking one.

References

Benson K and Hartz AJ (2000) A comparison of observational studies and randomized controlled trials. *NEJM*. **342**: 1878–86.

Concato J, Shah N and Horwitz RI (2000) Randomized controlled trials, observational studies and the hierarchy of research designs. *NEJM*. **342**: 1887–92.

Dosani S (2003) Practising medicine in a multicultural society. *BMJ*. **326**: s3–4.

Eliot TS (1944) *Four Quartets (Little Giddings)*. Faber and Faber, London.

Ewing AC (1951) *The Fundamental Questions of Philosophy*. Routledge & Kegan Paul, London.

Guthrie WKC (trans.) (1956) *The Meno*. Penguin, Harmondsworth.

Ogden J, Fuks K, Gardner M *et al.* (2002) Doctors' expressions of uncertainty and patient confidence. *Patient Education and Counselling*. **48**: 171–6.

Pocock SJ and Elbourne DR (2000) Randomized trials or observational tribulations. *NEJM*. **342**: 1907–9.

Thomas KB (1987) General practice consultations: is there any point in being positive? *BMJ*. **294**: 1200–2.

The nurse finished putting on the new dressing. The registrar sat up, feeling a little faint.

'Are you alright?', asked the elderly duty consultant, returning to the room. 'You are a little pale, you know.'

'I was on call last night. I haven't slept much for a couple of nights. I'll be fine, though. Thanks.'

'I see. It is rather tough, isn't it – these long shifts, not much sleep. Patients, patients, patients. Mind you, it was like that in my younger days, too. We had fewer things we could do – though in some ways that might have been a bit easier. But even old fossils like me still had penicillin and the sulphonamides when I started out in practice. Just imagine having no antibiotics at all, or – God help us – no practical anaesthesia apart from a blow to the head with a cushioned mallet or getting the patient blind drunk, or something similarly barbaric. Imagine dealing with profuse bleeding by cauterising with a heated iron or boiling oil. Hardly bears thinking about. Worked for some – didn't work for many others, though; if you didn't bleed to death then infection knocked you on the head.' She was silent for a moment, looking kindly at the registrar. 'You know, the basic problems in medicine are what they always were – pain, and sorrow.'

Then the consultant abruptly left the room in response to her pager's insistent bleep.

But hasn't Hippocrates said it all already …? Philosophy of medicine and changing traditions

Heikki S Vuorinen

Introduction

> … the science of medicine would never have been discovered nor, indeed, sought for, were there no need for it. If sick men fared just as well eating and drinking and living exactly as healthy men do, and no better on some different regimen, there would be little need for the science. But the reason why the art of medicine became necessary was because sick men did not get well on the same regimen as the healthy, any more than they do now.
>
> (Lloyd, 1978, p. 71)

This was how one Hippocratic author saw the origin of medicine. If we try to understand history by expecting it to have some practical use for a modern physician, there is a risk that we will see in it an inevitable progression from the darkness of superstitions and mistaken ideas to the light of modern, true science. Viewing history in that way, we tend to notice only those historical theories and practices which seem to herald modern ones. I hope the reader will keep this caveat in mind.

In this essay I have quite a modest aim, namely to provide the student of medicine with some idea of medical philosophy in the ancient world. For the ancient Greeks, medicine was a *techne* (art) which united theory with practical skills. To give an exhaustive presentation of the relationship between philosophy and medicine or medical philosophy during what is commonly called the Classical period is beyond the scope of this chapter. Ancient Greek (and to a lesser extent Roman) medicine has been the subject of innumerable books and articles in more recent times. The general features of the relationship between philosophy and medicine around the Mediterranean are well known for the period from the fifth century BC up to the fifth century AD, which roughly corresponds to the period in which we are interested. However, because the sources are in many ways defective, there is plenty of room for new interpretations. In this chapter I am going to consider the problems facing the ancient physician in the way in which a modern practitioner might conceive and distinguish them, namely in terms of the nature and causes of diseases, the sources of medical knowledge, diagnosis, the choice and implementation of treatments, and finally (though not least) ethical considerations.

The author of that part of the Hippocratic writings known as *Epidemics I* crystallised the challenges confronted by physicians throughout history:

> Consider what has gone before, recognise the signs before your eyes and then make your prognosis. Study these principles. Practice two things in your dealings with disease: either help or do not harm the patient. There are three factors in the practice of medicine: the disease, the patient and the physician. The physician is the servant of the science, and the patient must do what he can to fight the disease with the assistance of the physician.
>
> (Lloyd, 1978, pp. 93–4)

To understand how Western medicine originated in the ancient Greek world we must know the ailments for which people sought help from their healers, including their doctors (*iatroi*). Micro-organisms were by far the most serious threat to human health, and the evidence suggests that there were great secular and regional variations in the occurrence of diseases during antiquity. However, the sources do not enable us to estimate the frequency of a specific disease in different populations and time periods. Even so, we can safely assume that malaria in particular (including falciparum malaria) was widespread in the classical world, and that it had a definitive influence on the development of medicine (Jones, 1967).

Medicine in ancient Greece did not develop in a vacuum. We can trace at least two different roots for classical Greek medicine – first, the earlier advanced civilisations (Egypt and Mesopotamia), and secondly, traditional Greek popular medicine. The Greeks respected Egyptian medicine, while the Phoenician traders must have had an important role in conveying Mesopotamian ideas to the Greek world. However, Egyptian and Mesopotamian influences on Greek rational medicine have been considered to be minor, although they happened to share several characteristics with it

(Nutton, 1992; Longrigg, 1993). Traditional Greek popular medicine is not well known, because of the lack of sources.

Medical practitioners were almost exclusively men, and during the period of interest to us, most of them were Greeks. Social and economic conditions in the world around them changed considerably as time went on. The open, competitive society around the Aegean Sea in the fifth century BC changed to a world dominated by Hellenistic kingdoms, Carthage and the Roman Republic. The world of later antiquity became, in effect, a more or less centralised Roman Empire. The main problem inhibiting the development of medicine (and indeed sciences in general) was the lack of scientific organisations and institutions (Lloyd, 1983). The closest approach to a scientific institution in ancient times consisted of the Alexandrian Museum and Library during the era of the first Ptolemaic pharaohs (323–222 BC). During this relatively short period, the leading representatives of various disciplines, including medicine, were gathered together in Alexandria for the advancement of the sciences. The *Hippocratic Corpus*, the famous collection of Greek medical writings mainly composed around 400 BC, was brought together and collated in Alexandria. Indeed, Alexandria maintained its position as the leading centre of medicine until the Arabs conquered the city in the middle of seventh century AD.

A new medical institution, the hospital, developed during later antiquity, when Christianity secured a dominant position in the Roman world (Miller, 1985). We have very little knowledge of how this institution directly affected the practice of medicine, but it was plausibly an example of changing ethical responsibility in that society (Temkin, 1991).

The nature and causes of diseases

The so-called Ionian (Milesian) Natural Philosophers (Thales, Anaximenes and Anaximander) rejected any supernatural causes of natural phenomena as early as the sixth century BC (Lloyd, 1970). One of the early philosophers who particularly influenced ancient medical ideas was the Sicilian Empedocles (500–430 BC). Empedocles himself might even have been a physician. He developed the idea that everything which existed was composed of four elements – earth, fire, water and air. This idea, that there are just four basic elements, was to survive for over 2000 years. Empedocles (according to another scholar, Aëtius) considered the human body to be formed from mixtures of these elements:

> Empedocles says that flesh originates from the four elements mixed in equal proportions; sinews from fire and earth mixed with double the

amount of water; the claws of animals come into being from the sinews in so far as they happen to be chilled by contact with the air; bones from two parts of water and two of earth but four of fire, these parts being mixed with the earth. Sweat and tears come from blood as it dissolves and melts away according to its fluidity.

(Longrigg, 1998, p. 35)

Our knowledge of Greek medicine as such before the Hippocratic era is meagre. Pliny summed it up as follows: 'The subsequent story of medicine, strange to say, lay hidden in darkest night down to the Peloponnesian War, when it was restored to the light by Hippocrates (Jones, 1975, pp. 182–5). Indeed, among the few pre-Hippocratic Greek medical writers whose ideas have actually survived to our day, Alcmaeon of Croton from Southern Italy (who flourished around 470 BC, at roughly the same time as the Sicilian Empedocles) is the only one known to have studied the influence of Ionian Natural Philosophy on medicine. He adopted a cosmic theory as the basis of his own theory of health. Basically similar ideas were taken throughout antiquity to be essential parts of theories of health and disease. According to Aëtius:

Alcmaeon holds that what preserves health is the equality [*isonomia*] of the powers – moist and dry, cold and hot, bitter and sweet and the rest – and the supremacy [*monarchia*] of any one of them causes disease; for the supremacy of either is destructive. The cause of disease is an excess of heat or cold; the occasion of it surfeit or deficiency of nourishment; the location of it blood, marrow or the brain. Disease may come about from external causes, from the quality of water, local environment or toil or torture. Health, on the other hand, is a harmonious blending of the qualities.

(Longrigg, 1998, p. 31)

The greatest ancient philosophers, namely Plato (427–347 BC) and Aristotle (384–322 BC), adopted the theory of four basic elements. Plato was a younger contemporary of Hippocrates (who according to tradition lived c. 460–380 BC) and he knew the famous physician.[1] Indeed, Plato was generally well acquainted with medicine. His dialogue *Timaios* has been considered to be a synthesis of contemporary medical and philosophical knowledge (Nutton, 1992). In this dialogue Plato reviews (among other things) the parts of the body and the causes of diseases. It is not surprising that in a second-century AD medical papyrus known as *Anonymus Londinensis* the major part in the section considering the causes of diseases is devoted to Plato (Jones, 1947).

---

[1]Plato. *Protagoras* 311b, *Phaidros* 270c.

One may assume medicine's influence on the way in which Aristotle connected the four elements (fire, air, earth and water) to the four qualities (hot, cold, dry and wet). Aristotle came from a medical family and was extremely interested in biology, so it is not surprising that there are numerous observations on the medical profession and medicine in his works. Aristotle can also be regarded as the father of formal logic, and he concluded that the sciences could be presented as deductive systems. We can say without exaggeration that Aristotle's ideas have had an enduring influence on philosophy of medicine.

Later in antiquity the ideas of the basic constituents of the world around us, and knowledge of the basic structure of the human body, were developed into the theory of the four basic elements, the four humours and the four qualities (*see* Figure 1). This 'model' explaining the relationships between the world and human beings could also, and conveniently, be readily connected to the four seasons of the year and to the four constitutions (choleric, melancholic, phlegmatic and sanguine) of human beings.

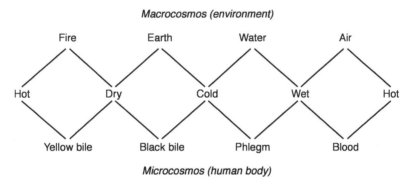

Figure 1 The way in which relationships between basic elements, qualities and humours have been traditionally expressed.

The materialistic philosopher Democritus (a contemporary of Hippocrates, who lived c. 460–370 BC) was, like Aristotle, greatly interested in biology and medicine. Unfortunately, only fragments of his ideas have survived, through the works of other authors. He seems to have had an influence on some of the authors of the *Hippocratic Corpus* and also later on the Methodist sect in medicine (Longrigg, 1993, pp. 66–9). Celsus's *De Medicina* preserved the tradition of a connection between Democritus and Hippocrates and the role that the latter had in distinguishing medicine from philosophy:

> Hence we find that many who professed philosophy became expert in medicine, the most celebrated being Pythagoras, Empedocles and

Democritus. But it was, as some believe, a pupil of the last, Hippo-crates of Cos ... who separated this branch of learning from the study of philosophy.

(Spencer, 1948, p. 5)

However, The *Hippocratic Corpus* clearly reveals that different physicians had different opinions of the relationship between medicine and philo-sophy, and Hippocrates' actual role in the separation of philosophy and medicine is not clearly settled (Jouanna, 1998).

One of the main achievements of ancient Greek medicine compared with earlier civilisations was the dismissal of supernatural causes of diseases in favour of an attempt at a rational understanding. An idea of nature as an ordered, regular, 'normal' phenomenon, that could be systematically observed and logically considered formed the basis of Hippocratic medicine. At the same time we must remember that the ancient Greek physicians were not atheists, and religion and medicine lived harmoniously together throughout Classical times. (It was only in the Christian Later Roman Empire that there began to be friction between medicine and the dominant religion) (Amundsen, 1996, pp. 127–74).

Some of the best examples of ideas of rational causation of diseases can be found in the Hippocratic treatise entitled *The Sacred Disease*. The author starts his brief monograph on epilepsy with the following words:

I do not believe that the 'Sacred Disease' is any more divine or sacred than any other disease but, on the contrary, has specific characteris-tics and a definite cause.

(Lloyd, 1978, p. 237)

Later he expresses this idea again:

I believe that this disease is not in the least more divine than any other, but has the same nature as other diseases and a similar cause. Moreover, it can be cured no less than other diseases, so long as it has not become inveterate and too powerful for the drugs which are given. Like other diseases it is hereditary.

(Lloyd, 1978, p. 240)

Finally the author concludes his ideas as follows:

This so-called 'sacred disease' is due to the same causes as all other diseases, to the things we see come and go, the cold and the sun, too, the changing and constant winds. These things are divine, so that there is no need to regard this disease as more divine than any other; all are alike divine and all human.

(Lloyd, 1978, p. 251)

The author of *The Sacred Disease* may also have been the author of at least some part of another famous Hippocratic treatise, entitled *Airs, Waters, Places*. Both of these writings belong to the early fourth century BC. *Airs, Waters, Places* recalls the position expressed in *The Sacred Disease*:

Indeed, I myself hold that this [impotence] and all other diseases are equally of divine origin and none more divine nor more earthly than another. Each disease has a natural cause, and nothing happens without a natural cause.

(Lloyd, 1978, p. 165)

Although these quotations exhibit rational thinking, we must always remember the huge differences between widespread beliefs in the ancient world and those in our own society. For instance, the idea that towns facing east are healthy (Lloyd, 1978, p. 151) and towns facing west are unhealthy (Lloyd, 1978, p. 151) may originate from Greek religious cults that considered east to be a clean direction and west to be an unclean one (Langholf, 1990). Prophesy also had an important place throughout antiquity. The important place of prognosis in ancient Greek medicine may thus resemble the status of religious augury or prophesy (Langholf, 1990, pp. 232–54).

Change was a very important philosophical concept in ancient medicine (Lloyd, 1970), nowhere more so than in conceptions of disease causation. Changing seasons were particularly important, but so also were changes in one's normal daily regimen of food, drink and exercise. Moreover, changes in the humoral composition of the human body led to diseases. However, change also had beneficial aspects – it was change that restored an ill person's health. In the words of a Hippocratic physician, 'the healthy person is not benefited by changes from his present state, but the ill one is' (Potter, 1995, p. 77) and 'everything that changes from the existing state benefits what is ill, for if you do not change what is ill, it increases' (Potter, 1995, p. 77)

Another important philosophical concept throughout ancient (and also later) medicine was moderation – the avoidance of extremes. In many Hippocratic works the process that causes disease is divided into external factors and the standard pathological processes in the human organism (*see* Figure 2).

The process leading from external causes to disease is lucidly described in the Hippocratic treatise *Affections*, traditionally dated to about 400 BC:

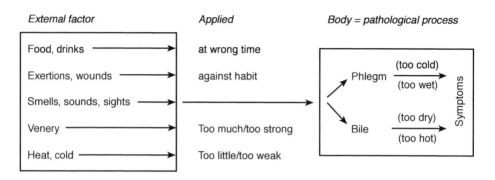

Figure 2   The process leading to diseases according to *Affections* 1, modified from Potter (1988c).

> ... all human diseases arise from bile and phlegm; the bile and phlegm produce diseases when, inside the body, one of them becomes too moist, too dry, too hot, or too cold; they become this way from foods and drinks, from exertions and wounds, from smell, sound, sight, and venery, and from heat and cold; this happens when any of the things mentioned are applied to the body at the wrong time, against custom, in too great amount and too strong, or in insufficient amount and too weak.
>
> (Potter, 1988a, p. 7)

This division is also seen throughout later antiquity, for instance in *Anonymus Londinensis*, a large part of which consists of a student's notes on that part of Menon's medical encyclopaedia which handles the causation of diseases. Menon was himself a follower of Aristotle. Most of the concepts of disease causation in *Anonymus Londinensis* (which presents the ideas of 19 ancient philosophers and physicians) are linked to nutrition and/or the four 'basic elements'. Pathological processes in the human body were explained using the theory of the four basic humours, which is why this theory is called humoralism or even humoral pathology (Nutton, 1993). The influence of the humors varied in Hippocratic writings, and it was not until Galen that a final synthesis of humoralism was achieved (*see* Figure 1). The humoral theory, which very economically explained the origin of diseases and their pathology, survived for over 2000 years as the basis of medical thinking.

Airs, Waters, Places includes some famous and often-quoted passages which show a close relationship between keen observation and rational, logical thinking on environmental (and social) causes of disease:

> Whoever would study medicine aright must learn of the following subjects. First, he must consider the effect of the seasons of the year

and the differences between them. Secondly, he must study the warm and the cold winds, both those that are common to every country and those peculiar to a particular locality. Lastly, the effect of water on the health must not be forgotten. Just as it varies in taste and when weighed, so does its effect on the body vary as well. When, therefore, a physician comes to a district previously unknown to him, he should consider both its situation and its aspects to winds. The effect of any town upon the health of its population varies according as it faces north or south, east or west. This is of the greatest impor-tance. Similarly, the nature of the water supply must be considered; is it marshy and soft, hard as it is when it flows from high and rocky ground, or salty with a hardness which is permanent? Then think of the soil, whether it be bare and waterless or thickly covered with vegetation and well-watered; whether in a hollow and stifling, or exposed and cold. Lastly, consider the life of the inhabitants themselves; are they heavy drinkers and eaters and consequently unable to stand fatigue or, being fond of work and exercise, eat wisely but drink sparely?

(Lloyd, 1978, p. 148)

The influence of seasons, climate and quality of water on the variation of diseases in a population in a particular location is the subject of lengthy discussion in *Airs, Waters, Places*, and the influence of the seasons also enjoyed a prominent place in many other Hippocratic writings.

The author of another Hippocratic writing *The Nature of Man*, reasoned philosophically, sharp-sightedly and logically, dividing the causes of diseases into two, namely the air that we breathe and the way of life that we follow.

Some diseases are produced by the manner of life that is followed; others by the life-giving air we breathe. That there are these two types may be demonstrated in the following way. When a large number of people all catch the same disease at the same time, the cause must be ascribed to something common to all and which they all use; in other words to what they all breathe. In such a disease, it is obvious that individual bodily habits cannot be responsible because the malady attacks one after another, young and old, men and women alike, those who drink their wine neat and those who drink only water; those who eat barley-cake as well as those who live on bread, those who take a lot of exercise and those who take but little. The regime cannot therefore be responsible where people who live very different lives catch the same disease. However, when many different diseases appear at the same time, it is plain that the regimen is responsible in individual cases. ... For, in such a case, it is obvious that all, most, or at least one of the factors in the regimen does not agree with the patient; such must be sought out and changed. ... When an epidemic of one particular disease is established, it is evident that it is not the regimen but the air breathed which is responsible. Plainly, the air must be harmful because of some morbid secretion which it contains.

(Lloyd, 1978, pp. 266–7)

For the preservation of one's health the author of *The Nature of Man* had sound practical advice, which was eagerly followed subsequently, especially in plague-stricken times, to arrange 'a change of station from the infected area'. The idea of the corruption of air was later developed into the idea of disease-causing miasma – a noxious change in the atmosphere arising from, for instance, the soil, water, sewers and especially decomposing organic matter. The miasma theory was very influential until as recently as the nineteenth century when, for instance, it formed the theoretical basis for the sanitation of British towns.

A person's way of life was considered to be a potential cause of disease in many Hippocratic writings, and later during antiquity by many medical and other authors. The preservation of one's health through a meticulous regime (of exercise, food and drink) was an important topic from then on. The recognition of the role of diet in the promotion of health and the prevention of diseases survived throughout the Middle Ages and up to modern times (Mikkeli, 1999).

Sources of medical knowledge

How did the ancient physician acquire knowledge of the nature and aetiology of diseases apart from logical reasoning? In many Hippocratic writings we clearly see the importance of detailed observations for ancient medicine. For instance, the seven volumes of *Epidemics* include hundreds of case histories, some of which are very detailed. However, the ancient physician did not pursue empirical studies in the modern sense (Lloyd, 1979; Langholf, 1990). Ancient doctors and other 'scientists' lacked (among other things) the concept of statistical probability, and this presented a significant obstacle to empirical studies (Lloyd, 1983). The Hippocratic physician also did not dissect human beings, so his knowledge of the internal structures of the human body was meagre.

A significant increase in medical knowledge occurred in Alexandria in Hellenistic times. Two fundamentally new ways of acquiring medical knowledge seem to have developed, namely dissecting the human body and conducting experiments. Unfortunately, no single intact work of the most famous early Alexandrian physicians Herophilus (who flourished around 300 BC) and Erasistratus (who was a little later than Herophilus) has survived to modern times. We know their opinions on medicine only from surviving fragments in the writings of later medical authors such as Galen. This lack of sources is really regrettable, as we can reasonably suppose that the philosophy of medicine in early Alexandria was much more versatile than is indicated by the short and partial sources that are actually available to us.

For a short period, the study of human anatomy by means of dissection was possible. In Greek culture there were strong taboos against dissecting human bodies, but in Alexandria under the protection of the first Ptolemaic pharaohs it was socially permissible to dissect human cadavers and probably also to vivisect criminals (Longrigg, 1993, pp. 184–90). Celsus in the first century AD wrote quite a lot about these methods of medical investigation:

> Moreover, as pains, and also various kinds of diseases, arise in the more internal parts, they [the Dogmatists] hold that no one can apply remedies for these who is ignorant about the parts themselves; hence it becomes necessary to lay open bodies of the dead and to scrutinise their viscera and intestines. They hold that Herophilus and Erasistratus did this in the best way by far, when they laid open men whilst alive – criminals received out of prison from the kings – and whilst these were still breathing, observed parts which beforehand nature had concealed, their position, colour, shape, size, arrangement, hardness, softness, smoothness, relation, processes and depressions of each, and whether any part is inserted into or received into another. For when pain occurs internally, neither is it possible for one to learn what hurts the patient, unless he has acquainted himself with the position of each organ or intestine; nor can a diseased portion of the body be treated by one who does not know what that portion is. When a man's viscera are exposed in a wound, he who is ignorant of the colour of a part in health may be unable to recognise which part is intact, and which part damaged; thus he cannot even relieve the damaged part. External remedies too can be applied more aptly by one acquainted with the position, shape and size of the internal organs, and like reasoning hold good in all the instances mentioned above. Nor is it, as most people say, cruel that in the execution of criminals, and but a few of them, we should seek remedies for innocent people of all future ages.
>
> (Spencer, 1948, pp. 12–15)

Unlike the Dogmatists whose views he rehearses here, Celsus was himself hostile to vivisection. However, he clearly approved the general principle of dissection when studying medicine:

> Therefore, to return to what I myself propound, I am of the opinion that the Art of Medicine ought to be rational, but to draw instruction from evident causes, all obscure ones being rejected from the practice of the Art, although not from the practitioner's study. But to lay open the bodies of men whilst still alive is as cruel as it is needless; that of the dead is a necessity for learners, who should know positions and relations, which the dead body exhibits better than does a living and wounded man. As for the remainder, which can only be learnt from the living, actual practice will demonstrate it in the course of treating the wounded in a somewhat slower yet much milder way.
>
> (Spencer, 1948, p. 41)

These arguments on the part of the Dogmatists – and of Celsus himself – for and against particular research methods sound quite familiar in modern medicine. This period of fervent anatomical studies was short. After the end of the early Alexandrian period the medical student in antiquity had to rely an animal dissections, skeletinised cadavers and wounded gladiators, soldiers, and so on (Lloyd, 1979; Longrigg, 1993, pp. 218–19). The rapid increase in anatomical vocabulary during the Hellenic period is almost anarchic in its character. This in itself shows clearly how the lack of unifying institutions, as well as the harsh competition between different types of medical practitioners, placed significant obstacles in the way of the accumulation of medical knowledge (Lloyd, 1983, pp. 165–6).

According to later tradition, it seems that Erasistratus might have concluded experimental studies:

> In addition to all this, Erasistratus too attempts to establish the point thus. If one were to take a creature, such as a bird or something of the sort, and were to place it in a pot for some time without giving it any food, and then were to weigh it with the excrement that visibly has been passed, he will find that there has been a great loss of weight, plainly because, perceptible only to the reason, a copious emanation has taken place.
>
> (Jones, 1947, pp. 126–7)

If we knew more about these early Alexandrian physicians, we might form quite different opinions about the role of experimental studies during antiquity (Lloyd, 1979, pp. 223–4).

Several medical sects (e.g. Empiricists, Dogmatists, Methodists, Pneumatists, Herophileans and Erasistrateans) developed during the Hellenistic and Roman periods. These sects differed in (among other things) their opinions on the correct method in medicine. Dogmatists were happy to speculate about 'hidden causes' and argued that knowledge of the constitution of man (including anatomy) and the causes of diseases was essential to medical practice. Empiricists, in contrast, argued that such speculations are neither legitimate nor necessary. For the Empiricist the physician's task was to treat individual cases and to be guided only by the manifest symptoms of the patient and earlier experience. The Empiricists, according to Celsus, thus explicitly dissociated themselves from philosophers:

> On the other hand, those who are called 'Empirici' because they have experience do indeed accept evident causes as necessary; but they contend that inquiry about obscure causes and natural actions is superfluous, because nature is not to be comprehended. That nature cannot be comprehended is in fact patent, they say, from the disagreement among those who discuss such matters; for on this question there is no agreement, either among professors of philosophy or among actual medical practitioners. ... Even philosophers would have become the greatest of medical practitioners, if reasoning from theory could have made them so; as it is, they have words in plenty, and no knowledge of healing at all ... that if the evident cause does not supply the knowledge, much less can a cause which is in doubt yield it. Since, therefore, the cause is as uncertain as it is incomprehensible, protection is to be sought rather from the ascertained and explored, as in all the rest of the Arts, that is, from what experience has taught in the actual course of treatment.
>
> (Spencer, 1948, pp. 15–17)

During the Roman period there were several medical authors whose works have survived until modern times. The most famous of these is Galen (c. 130–200 AD) (Nutton 1996; Gourevitch, 1998). That proportion of his writings which has survived to the present day is itself twice as large as the *Hippocratic Corpus*. An appreciable part of Galen's work consists of commentaries on Hippocratic treatises. We might say that Galen was the person who finally elevated Hippocrates to the status of 'the father of medicine' (although Galen was not a modest man, considering himself to be second only to Hippocrates among physicians). Another group of Galen's works consists of textbooks for medical students and medical handbooks.

Galen emphasised the role of philosophy for physicians. His philosophical ideas originate mainly from Aristotle, but also from Plato and the Stoics.

However, his role as an original philosopher has become more widely appreciated in recent decades. Galen stressed the importance of logical reasoning in medicine. He was interested in the problem of causation of diseases and the influence of the environment on people's health. His importance in broadening medical knowledge is well demonstrated in anatomy. Although Galen probably only dissected animals, he was able to correct earlier ideas. For instance, he showed that arteries are always full of blood, and thereby refuted the older view that they contained nothing but air. His work shows how some accumulation of medical knowledge did indeed take place during antiquity, despite the many obstacles in its path.

Diagnosis and prognosis

What did an ancient physician do when a person came to seek help for some ailment or injury? First of all he had to recognise what type of disease was involved. It took a keen observer to note, as the ancient physician did indeed do, every detail of the condition of the patient with the help of all his senses. 'The task is to bring the body under consideration. Vision, hearing, nose, touch, tongue, reasoning arrive at knowledge' (Smith, 1994, p. 285, pp. 137–9; Withington, 1948, p. 59). The physician used his hands to palpate the patient's abdomen and the vessels (Potter, 1995, pp. 227, 269). Some of the Hippocratic physicians also used direct auscultation in the case of lung or chest ailments, sometimes shaking the patient while listening to them (Potter 1988a, pp. 273–5, 303, 307; Potter, 1988b, p. 53; Potter, 1995, p. 55). When examining wounds, fistulas, etc, different types of probes or mirrors were used. If the physician was uncertain of his diagnosis (or prognosis), the patient could be strenuously exercised if the signs of disease were not observable at rest. Alternatively, certain foods or preparations were administered in order to produce the relevant signs.

> Even when nature herself does not produce such signs, they may be revealed by certain harmless measures known to those practised in the science.... Thus a visible sign is produced of some underlying disease, which could not otherwise be demonstrated to the sight. If a patient be made to walk uphill or to run, abnormalities in respiration will be observed which would not be apparent at rest.
>
> (Lloyd, 1978, p. 147)

The Hippocratic physician accurately recorded the symptoms of the patient. However, he was not so focused on the diagnosis as his modern colleague is. There might even have been differences between various schools of medicine with regard to the importance of diagnosis as such

(Lloyd, 1978, p. 186), and the development of the nosology of diseases is traditionally associated with only the medical 'school' on the island of Cnidus (Jouanna, 1998).

By contrast, the near universal importance of the *prognosis* in medicine might have something to do with the heavy competition between different groups of healers in the ancient world:

> It seems to be highly desirable that a physician should pay much attention to prognosis. If he is able to tell his patients when he visits them not only about their past and present symptoms, but also to tell them what is going to happen, as well as to fill in the details they have omitted, he will increase his reputation as a medical practitioner, and people will have no qualms in putting themselves under his care. Moreover, he will the better be able to effect a cure if he can foretell, from the present symptoms, the future course of the disease. It is impossible to cure all patients; that would be an achievement surpassing in difficulty even the forecasting of future developments. ... One must know to what extent they [diseases] exceed the strength of the body, and one must have a thorough acquaintance with their future course. In this way one may become a good physician and justly win high fame. In the case of patients who were going to survive, he would be able to safeguard them the better from complications by having a longer time to take precautions. By realising and announcing beforehand which patients were going to die, he would absolve himself from any blame.
>
> (Lloyd, 1978, p. 170)

A medical sect in those days had no way of compelling its own members – for less all other physicians – to follow a common set of ideas. Fervent competition between and within different groups of healers characterised the Mediterranean world in antiquity. The open, competitive society around the Aegean Sea in the fifth century BC seems to have been especially fruitful for the development of philosophy and medicine as witnessed by the Hippocratic writings (Nutton, 1992). In this environment it was obviously essential to develop logical thinking and consistent theories in medicine. Furthermore, because medical practitioners generally lacked quick and efficient remedies or cures, it must have been easier to triumph over rival practitioners in philosophical debate than in medical practice!

Medical treatments

In practice, most ancient physicians probably followed more or less closely the teachings of the Empirics, treating their patients on the basis of experience without much philosophical speculation. They had four principal forms of treatment, namely a prescribed regimen (diet, exercise, and so on), drugs, surgery and cauterisation. The Hippocratic authors recommended caution in the use of these treatments (Lloyd, 1978, pp. 208–9, 212; Jouanna, 1998, pp. 193–7; Potter, 1995, p. 77), and in the sixth book of *Epidemics* there is the famous statement that nature heals (Potter, 1995, p. 255). The general condition of the patient was considered to be important, so that for instance healthy, sick and convalescent people were regarded as needing different kinds of regimen.

Some physicians were quite confident of their abilities to help their patients:

> Each has its own nature and character, and there is nothing in any disease which is unintelligible or which is insusceptible to treatment. The majority of maladies may be cured by the same things as caused them. ... A man with the knowledge of how to produce by means of a regimen dryness and moisture, cold and heat in the human body, could cure this disease [epilepsy] too, provided that he could distinguish the right moment for the application of the remedies. He would not need to resort to purifications and magic spells.
>
> (Lloyd, 1978, p. 251)

This therapeutic optimism expressed by the author of *The Sacred Disease* stands in contrast to remarks advising the physician to be careful to distinguish those diseases that can be treated from those that cannot (Potter, 1988a, p. 113). However, this contrast may appear to be more imaginary than real if we emphasise the words 'provided that he could distinguish the right moment'. The overall spirit of Hippocratic writings favours the active treatment of every patient, while recognising that in many cases the treatment is merely palliative.

Plato was perhaps the most influential ancient author to be frankly sceptical about the use of drugs. He even considered interference in the ordinary progress of the disease and the use of drugs to be dangerous for the patient:

> ... and so he will not leave foe ranged by foe to produce conflict and disease in the body, but friend by friend to produce health. Among movements, the best is that we produce in ourselves of ourselves – for it is most nearly akin to the movement of thought and of the universe. ... So the best way of purging and toning up the body is by exercise ... last, and for use in extreme necessity, though not otherwise if we have any sense, is purging by medicine and drugs. Indeed, unless the danger is grave, diseases should not be irritated by drugs.

For the course of a disease resembles the life of an animal ... and if their allotted period is interfered [with] by drugs, they are commonly rendered more serious or more frequent. All kinds of diseases therefore should, so far as leisure permits, be controlled by a proper regime of life, and stubborn complaints should not be irritated by drugs.

(Lee, 1987, p. 120)

Medicine in antiquity was an open science and practice, in sharp contrast to the working climate of the present medical profession. Laymen in antiquity could (and did) read medical treatises and practise medicine. The Hippocratic author of *Affections* addressed his work to laymen (although the target group was probably physicians):

Any man who is intelligent must, on considering that health is of the utmost value to human beings, have the personal understanding necessary to help himself in diseases, and be able to understand and to judge what physicians say and what they administer to his body, being versed in each of these matters to a degree reasonable for a layman ... let the layman be able to contribute an opinion with a certain amount of judgement.

(Potter, 1988a, pp. 7–9)

Later the author adds: 'Through understanding these things, a layman will be less likely to fall into incurable diseases that tend, from minor provocations, to become serious and chronic.' (Potter, 1988a, p. 57) Like Plato, some medical laymen were distinguished in other fields. The famous historian Thucydides (fifth century BC) was well acquainted with medicine (Jouanna, 1998), and almost 800 years later another soldier and historian, Ammianus Marcellinus, showed a considerable knowledge of medicine when, for instance, he described an epidemic in Amida (Syria) in 359 AD (Hamilton, 1986, pp. 167–8).

However, some distinction between professional and layman in medicine was clearly discernible even in antiquity. For instance, Aristotle clearly supported the role of medicine as a specific field of scientific knowledge and practice. He pondered the problem of the specific and the general in theory and practice, using medicine as an example:

Moreover, individual tuition, like individual treatment in medicine, is actually superior to the public sort. For example, as a general rule rest and fasting are beneficial in a case of fever, but not, perhaps, for a particular patient ... . It would seem, then, that particular cases receive more accurate treatment when individual attention is given, because then each person is more likely to get what suits him. But the best detailed treatment will be given by the doctor ... who has a general knowledge of what is good for all cases, or for a specific type; because the sciences not only are said to be but are concerned with common facts. This is not to deny that in a particular case it is probably quite possible for the right treatment to be given by one who has no knowledge, but has carefully observed (in the course of his experience) the effects upon individuals [of different kinds of treatment]; just as some people really seem to be their own best doctors, although they would be quite unable to help anybody else. Nevertheless, it would presumably be agreed that anyone who wants to be professionally qualified with theoretical knowledge must proceed to the study of the universal and get to know it as well as possible; for it is with this (as we have said) that the sciences deal ... . If anyone can do it, it is the man with knowledge – just as in the case of medicine and all the other professions that call for application and practical understanding ... . We do not find people becoming qualified in medicine by reading handbooks, although the authors at least attempt to describe ... general methods of treatment for each type of patient, classifying them by their [bodily] states; and these handbooks are considered to be helpful to the experienced, but useless to the layman.

(Thomson, 1987, pp. 339–41)

Medical ethics

The ancient physician had only a limited number of effective means for preventing diseases or caring for or curing his patients. Consequently, unlimited competition in the medical marketplace was the principal factor underlying the formation of the medical ethics of the time – itself one of classical medicine's significant achievements. It is quite likely that written ethical codes considerably enhanced patients' trust in their doctors, and of course this in turn increased the effectiveness of many medical treatments. Although some of the subjects within ancient medical ethics seem irrelevant to the modern practitioner (such as those parts that forbid surgery or determine the frames of medical training), many others are highly relevant even today, dealing with (among other things) the patient–doctor relationship, abortion, euthanasia and professional collegiality.

The *Hippocratic Corpus* includes several ethical works, namely *Oath*, *Precepts*, *Physician*, *Law* and *Decorum*. Perhaps the Hippocratic Oath is most familiar to modern physicians, although many of them may not know or remember its exact contents. However, other classical authors, including Plato, Aristotle, Celsus, Pliny, Soranos and Galen, also had much to say about medical ethics. For instance, Aristotle refers to medicine, physicians, health and sickness in several places in his famous *Nicomachean Ethics* (Thomson, 1987). However, as even a superficial examination of the social context of ancient medical ethics shows, there was no uniform system of medical ethics during antiquity. The anonymous Hippocratic physicians crystallised one of the enduring bases of ethical medical practice in this way, recorded by the author of the first book of *Epidemics*: 'Regarding diseases, make a practice of two things – to help, or, at least, to do no harm.' Later that writer clearly defined the roles of the doctor and the patient in the healing process:

> The art has three factors, the disease, the patient, and the doctor. The doctor is the servant of the art. The patient must co-operate with the doctor in combating the disease.
>
> (Lloyd, 1978, p. 94)

The Hippocratic Oath has undoubtedly been the most influential medical writing on ethics to survive from classical times. Generation after generation of physicians in the Western world has become familiarised with it during their education. The just and equal treatment of every human being is one of the basic tenets in this writing, which has retained its value to the present day:

> ... I will use treatments for the benefit of the sick to the best of my ability and judgement; I will abstain from doing harm or wronging any man by it .... Into whatsoever house I enter, I will enter for the benefit of the sick. I will abstain from all voluntary wrong-doing and harm, and especially from sexual contacts with the bodies of women or of men, whether free or slaves.
>
> (Longrigg, 1998, p. 101)

Let us give the last word to that Hippocratic author, who – echoing ideas expressed by Aristotle in his *Nicomachean Ethics* and *Politics* (Thomson, 1987, pp. 171–202), urging that the goal of medicine consists of producing health, and not the gathering of riches – advised physicians not to seek financial reward as their goal:

> One ought not, then, to be concerned about fixing a fee. For I consider an anxiety of this sort harmful to a troubled patient, much more so in the case of an acute disease .... It is better, therefore, to reproach patients whom you have saved than to extort money from those who are in a critical condition .... I recommend that you do not display overmuch incivility, but have regard to your patient's

means or wealth. On occasion give your services free ... for where there is love of man, there is also love of the art. For some sick people, though aware that their condition is dangerous, simply by being well-pleased with the goodness of their doctor, take a turn for the better.

(Longrigg, 1998, pp. 104–5)

References

Amundsen DW (1996) *Medicine, Society and Faith in the Ancient and Medieval Worlds.* The Johns Hopkins University Press, Baltimore, MD.

Gourevitch D (1998) The paths of knowledge: medicine in the Roman world. In: MD Grmek (ed.) *Western Medical Thought from Antiquity to the Middle Ages.* Harvard University Press, Cambridge, MA.

Hamilton W (1986) *Ammianus Marcellinus. The Later Roman Empire (AD 354–378).* Penguin, Harmondsworth.

Jones WHS (1947) *The Medical Writings of Anonymus Londinensis.* Cambridge University Press, Cambridge.

Jones WHS (1967) The prevalence of malaria in Ancient Greece. In: D Brothwell and AT Sandison (eds) *Diseases in Antiquity. A survey of the diseases, injuries and surgery of early populations.* Charles C Thomas, Springfield, IL.

Jones WHS (1975) *Pliny Natural History with an English Translation in Ten Volumes. Volume VIII. Libri XXVIII–XXXII.* The Loeb Classical Library, Harvard University Press, Cambridge, MA.

Jouanna J (1998) The birth of Western medical art. In: MD Grmek (ed.) *Western Medical Thought from Antiquity to the Middle Ages.* Harvard University Press, Cambridge, MA.

Langholf V (1990) *Medical Theories in Hippocrates. Early texts and the 'epidemics'.* Walter de Gruyter, Berlin.

Lee D (1987) *Plato. Timaeus and Critias.* Penguin Books, Harmondsworth.

Lloyd GER (1970) *Early Greek Science. Thales to Aristotle.* Chatto & Windus, London.

Lloyd GER (1979) *Magic, Reason and Experience. Studies in the origins and development of Greek science.* Cambridge University Press, Cambridge.

Lloyd GER (1983) *Science, Folklore and Ideology. Studies in the life sciences in Ancient Greece.* Cambridge University Press, Cambridge.

Lloyd GER (ed.) (1978) *Hippocratic Writings.* Penguin, Harmondsworth.

Longrigg J (1993) *Greek Rational Medicine. Philosophy and medicine from Alcmaeon to the Alexandrians.* Routledge, London.

Longrigg J (1998) *Greek Medicine. From the Heroic to the Hellenistic Age. A source book.* Duckworth, London.

Mikkeli H (1999) *Hygiene in the Early Modern Medical Tradition.* Annales Academiæ Scientiarum Fennicæ, Saarijärvi.

Miller TS (1985) *The Birth of the Hospital in the Byzantine Empire.* The Johns Hopkins University Press, Baltimore, MD.

Nutton V (1992) Healers in the medical marketplace: towards a social history of Graeco-Roman medicine. In: A Wear (ed.) *Medicine in Society. Historical essays.* Cambridge University Press, Cambridge.

Nutton V (1993) Humoralism. In: WF Bynum and R Porter (eds) *Companion Encyclopedia of the History of Medicine. Volume 1.* Routledge, London, pp. 6–11.

Nutton V (1996) Roman medicine, 250 BC to AD 200. In: LI Conrad, M Neve, V Nutton *et al.* (eds) *The Western Medical Tradition 800 BC to AD 1800.* Cambridge University Press, Cambridge.

Potter P (ed.) (1988a) *Hippocrates, Volume V.* The Loeb Classical Library, Harvard University Press, Cambridge, MA.

Potter P (ed.) (1988b) *Hippocrates. Volume VI.* The Loeb Classical Library, Harvard University Press, Cambridge, MA.

Potter P (1988c) *Short Handbook of Hippocratic Medicine.* Les Éditions du Sphinx, Québec.

Potter P (ed.) (1995) *Hippocrates. Volume VIII.* The Loeb Classical Library, Harvard University Press, Cambridge, MA.

Smith WD (ed.) (1994) *Hippocrates. Volume VII.* The Loeb Classical Library, Harvard University Press, Cambridge, MA.

Spencer WG (1948) *Celsus. De Medicina in Three Volumes. Volume I.* The Loeb Classical Library, Harvard University Press, Cambridge, MA.

Temkin O (1991) *Hippocrates in a World of Pagans and Christians.* The Johns Hopkins University Press, Baltimore, MD.

Thomson JAK (trans.) (1987) *The Ethics of Aristotle. The Nicomachean Ethics.* Penguin, Harmondsworth.

Withington ET (ed.) (1948) In the surgery 1. In: *Hippocrates. Volume III.* The Loeb Classical Library, Harvard University Press, Cambridge, MA.

The Chair of Surgery passed along the corridor and stopped at the open door.

'Ah, I heard about your accident. I'm sorry now that I invited you to do that appendectomy instead of looking after the ward patients this morning.'

'Sorry, Prof, this is really embarrassing.'

The registrar explained in some detail the events at the start of the operation. The Chair of Surgery nodded sympathetically.

'Don't worry about the patient's blood – I checked the records myself. You're fine on that score; nothing to worry about in terms of infection. By the way – I assume you've had your own antibody-check recently? Yes? Good. Here, are you really all right? You look like you've been awake for a week.'

'I pretty well have. Well, three days anyway.'

'When you feel up to driving home, go there at once, and take a week off. Then just see outpatients for a couple of weeks until your hand has recovered properly. This is for your own good – but for your patients' good as well, right? I know you're dedicated, and wanting to impress. But for pity's sake, these long hours aren't really helping anyone. This doctoring business isn't about heroics. It's about taking care of people. Agreed?'

'Agreed.'

'Yourself included.'

But who can say what's right and wrong? Medicine as a moral enterprise

Pekka Louhiala

Introduction

Abortion, cloning, informed consent, involuntary treatment, surrogate motherhood, euthanasia, rationing – these are examples which most people would probably suggest if they were asked to name some of the issues with which the subject of 'medical ethics' is usually concerned. I doubt whether such complaints as the common cold or simple ear infections would be mentioned at all. However, medicine is a *moral* enterprise in a very deep sense – probably every judgement that a physician makes involves both a factual and a moral judgement.

In this chapter I shall first demonstrate this moral dimension in the light of an ordinary everyday example – a child presenting with symptoms of a middle-ear infection. Then, I shall briefly review the types of intuitive answers that people give when they are faced with a moral problem, and I shall review how these answers reflect some of the major ethical theories that have been presented in the history of philosophical writing on morality. In the last part of the chapter I shall discuss the role that philosophy and philosophers could play in practical medical ethics.

The ethics of middle-ear infection

A two-year-old boy has had symptoms of the common cold for a couple of days. He wakes up in the middle of the night crying and complaining of pain in his left ear. He has a rising temperature and a mild fever.

On the face of it, the case seems obvious. Every medical practitioner, and indeed most parents, would suspect a middle-ear infection, which is the commonest complication of the common cold. From the point of view of medical decision making, the case may also seem to be simple. The little boy either has the infection or he does not have it – if he has it, then he will receive treatment based on evidence from clinical and basic research.

In real life, however, even in a simple case like this there are many steps at which not only judgements of fact but also *value judgements* are made. There are rather more of these value judgements than one might readily assume.

First, the process of *diagnosis* involves judgements that are not simply factual. There may be physical obstacles that prevent the doctor from looking at the tympanic membrane. The commonest of these is earwax, and removing it is often far from easy. In medical school we were taught that visualising the tympanic membrane is essential for making a diagnosis. Later on, though, medical practice showed us that very often we have to make a value judgement in a case like this. Does the certainty of the diagnosis outweigh the discomfort caused to the child when one is trying to remove the wax? As many practitioners know, this discomfort may sometimes be significant. Moreover, the business of making a reliable diagnosis is not helped by the fact that there are numerous definitions of middle-ear infection.

Secondly, decisions about *treatment* also involve value judgements. When the diagnosis is obvious, the first question that occurs to most doctors and parents is likely to be whether the little boy needs antibiotics or not. If he happens to live in Finland, he will probably be prescribed them, but if he lives in the Netherlands, his family doctor may well choose the 'wait-and-see' option – even when both the Finnish and Dutch doctors are aware of research (specifically, meta-analyses of drug trials) which suggests that we need to treat seven children with antibiotics if we are to expect that a single one of them will benefit as a result. These two doctors choose differently because their medical traditions are different. Evidence-based medicine gives us numbers and relationships between numbers (and in this case the NNT, the *number needed to treat*, is seven), but it becomes blind and numb when the final decision about treatment has to be made. This decision is again a *value* judgment. In a more dramatic case with the same NNT, but where the treatment in question was potentially a life-saving intervention (e.g. drug medication for an allergic reaction), no doctor would choose simply to 'wait and see'. Yet in the case of middle-ear infection many would do so.

If the doctor in charge chooses to prescribe antibiotics for the child, there are still several value judgments to be made, such as the choice of drug. Do the price, taste, number of daily doses or length of the course matter? If every dose means a struggle between the child and his parents, then the parents might well prefer a single daily dose for three days to a twice daily dose for a week. Should the drug have a wide antibiotic spectrum, or would a narrow spectrum be sufficient? In answering the last question the doctor has to balance the interests of the patient with those of society in general. Liberal use of wide-spectrum antibiotics may well increase the likelihood that a *present* intervention will be effective, but by increasing bacterial resistance to drugs such liberal use will very probably be harmful to many *future* patients.

There are other issues about treatment, too. Personally, I typically recommend an upright sleeping position for children with this condition, but this is based not on evidence-based medicine but on common sense. Again, strangely enough there is hardly any evidence to show any advantage from prescribing pain-relieving medication in the symptomatic treatment of these children. Despite this, my personal values suggest to me that it would be irresponsible and unethical *not* to recommend pain relief.

Thirdly, even after these treatment decisions we still face some further issues involving values. Does the child need a re-examination after a few weeks as the current Finnish recommendations suggest (without, by the way, any evidence of benefit)? Is it the doctor's business to ask about, or to comment upon, domestic issues that might help to prevent further morbidity (e.g. day-care arrangements or smoking in the family)? How should the doctor evaluate the surgical removal of adenoids after several episodes of middle-ear infection? In my own practice I often recommend the procedure *despite* the evidence suggested by clinical trials. This is because my clinical experience suggests that most children with recurrent middle-ear infections actually do benefit greatly from this operation. I am, of course, painfully aware of the fact that clinical experience can be very misleading.

This example of a child with a probable middle-ear infection does not involve questions of life and death in the way that many more 'high-profile' medical ethics questions do. Even so, it demonstrates that values and value judgements are woven into all medical practice – not only in the dramatic illnesses, but also in the very simple cases that are the daily bread of every physician.

From the middle ear to the muddle of ethical theory

It is typical of philosophy and philosophers that, among the issues which interest them, there are few on which we could find general agreement.

And just as for philosophical enquiry as a whole, so too for moral philosophy and moral philosophers – there seem to be many schools of thought, each of which emphasises different types of considerations as the basis of moral thinking. In the moral decisions of everyday life we do not usually contemplate deep philosophical questions but rather we make our judgements fairly intuitively. However, this does not mean that our everyday thinking is theory-free. On the contrary, fragments of major theories of moral philosophy can be traced in our thinking, although we are not usually aware of this.

Again, the case of middle-ear infection may illustrate this. On graduating from medical school I felt very strongly that my *duty* was to reach as certain a diagnosis as possible, otherwise I would not be acting in the way that a good doctor should. Sometimes this meant half an hour's work – after which three people (the child, the mother and myself) were bathed in perspiration. Thus it might be argued that the child's *rights* (to comfort, integrity, etc.) were violated without a sufficiently good reason. My own reasoning, when I make treatment decisions, includes comparing the *outcomes* of different options, (e.g. antibiotics or not). Now I have italicised three particular words in this paragraph because they point to philosophical theories in our everyday thinking.

First, we might refer to *duty*. The basic question in moral theories that are grounded on the idea of duty is 'What ought we to do?' (O'Neill, 1991). The frame of reference for identifying duties may be theological (religious) or it may be secular. Some examples of general rules referring to duty include the so-called golden rule ('do unto others as you would have them do unto you') in a Scriptural context (Matthew 7;12), and Immanuel Kant's *Categorical Imperative* ('act only on the maxim through which you can at the same time will that it be a universal law') in a secular context. The proponents of duty-based ethical theories argue from these very general rules towards their more specific and differentiated implementation. The main difficulties with this approach lie in tracing the route from the general to the particular (O'Neill, 1991). For example, in the medical context a very common ethical problem is that the patient does want what the doctor would want for herself in a similar situation, and thus does not want to be 'done unto' in the way that the doctor would have someone else do unto her – the golden rule simply does not help.

Secondly, the starting point in ethics may be *rights*. The *Oxford Companion to Philosophy* defines rights as follows: 'In their strongest sense, rights are justified claims to the protection of a person's important interests' (Honderich 1995). However, this definition seems to imply that if I have a right to X, there must be someone or something whose duty it is to make sure that I can actually have X. Of course, this is a simplified description of a right, and other types of rights can also be thought of. In the context of medicine and healthcare (and politics, for that matter), perhaps the important and most widely discussed right has been the right to self-determination, or autonomy as it is now more familiarly known. Respect for autonomy, and its opposite, paternalism, have often been presented dichotomously, in simple black-and-white terms – the former being offered as good and desirable and the latter as bad and undesirable. However, in real life there is a grey area between these two extremes, and it is often simply not possible to respect fully the autonomy of everyone who is party to a given situation, (e.g. if two or more of them have competing interests or wishes).

Thirdly, the basis of ethics might be the consequences or *outcomes* of our deeds. In our opening example, the doctor has to compare the probable outcomes of two treatment options – or as it is sometimes put, he weighs the 'utility' of these options. The school of philosophy which takes these 'utilities' as its starting point is called utilitarianism. The famous slogan about pursuing 'the greatest happiness of the greatest number' describes the basic idea. Cost–benefit calculations are an example of attempted utilitarian thinking in healthcare provision.

A fourth school of ethics is *virtue* ethics. I did not mention 'virtues' as such in our example, but I did refer to my striving to be a 'good doctor'. If we are satisfied with the way in which a professional does his or her work, we do not usually talk about their virtues – we simply refer to them as performing well. However, their personal, professional and moral virtues are implicit in this. Theories of 'virtue ethics' hold that morality cannot be reduced to a calculus of the harms and benefits of an action, or to universal claims against others. Instead, it pays attention to the particularities of individuals and cases (O'Neill, 1991).

Talking in a few short paragraphs about four major schools of moral philosophy is, of course, a gross over-simplification of thousands of years of scholarship. I wanted simply to demonstrate that our intuitive moral thinking, in medicine or elsewhere, is by no means disconnected from theory. Our intuitions have the same roots as do the various theoretical systems that have been developed in philosophy. Indeed, in our daily talk we do actually use terms like 'duty' and 'right', and we also refer to the consequences of our moral choices. Perhaps we do not use the term 'virtue' quite so often, but we do refer to the characteristics of a 'good doctor', a 'good nurse', a 'good citizen', and so on. Philosophers have written large volumes about these same issues, using the same terms, and trying to find the foundations of moral thinking.

Whose business is it anyway?

For a very long time the medical profession seemed to think that medical ethics belonged to medicine and to medicine alone. What is more, the public did not disagree with this to any great extent. Philosophical ethics of the early twentieth century were rather theoretical, and were not much interested in medicine or medical ethics. However, the latter part of the century did finally bring philosophers into the arena of medical ethics. There were three main reasons for this involvement.

First, technological developments in medicine after the Second World War had created apparently new ethical problems, without any obvious historical precedent. In particular, the development of intensive care and organ transplantation in the 1960s brought about challenges which launched a co-operation between medical doctors, moral philosophers and moral theologians. Then it soon became obvious that medical expertise as such does not include or entail expertise in moral issues. Developments in other areas of medical science and practice, such as reproductive medicine in the 1970s and genetics in the 1980s, created further challenges to be dealt with. There seems to be no end to this development, as new instances of ethical problems in medicine emerge every year. Even where no new *kind* of challenge is apparent, such development continually gives us new instances, applications or contexts of challenges with which we think we have become familiar. (In a nutshell, when science gives us the physical ability to do something new, does it follow from this that we ought to attempt it? Answering this question is not in itself a scientific matter.)

Secondly, the rise of political individualism in many areas of life was strongly reflected in the practice of medicine. Doctors' standing and position 'next to God' became more and more questionable, and people's right to determine matters that affected their own lives became more obvious. Philosophers had a role in this development, when some of them stressed autonomy as a key value in medical ethics (however, not all agree, and some philosophers have heavily criticised the dominance of patient autonomy within medical ethics discussions) (Welie, 1998).

Thirdly, the success of biologically oriented medicine or *biomedicine* was substantial, yet still it was unable to solve the world's major health problems. The wellbeing of people was not directly related to something that could be scientifically measured. First medical ethics, and later more generally philosophy of medicine, were called upon for help in addressing the 'identity crisis' of clinical medicine. The involvement of philosophers and philosophy in medicine grew rapidly during the 1970s and 1980s, and the academic disciplines of philosophical medical ethics and bioethics were established. Some philosophers began to call themselves 'bioethicists' and (particularly in the USA) 'clinical ethicists'. The latter give consultations in ethical problems in much the same way that specialists in medical subdisciplines give consultations in their own areas of expertise.

We saw above that philosophers do not even agree about the foundations on which ethics should be built. Can they then contribute in a meaningful way to solving the very practical problems that are encountered in real-life medical ethics?

If we are looking for simple answers or directives, the obvious answer is 'No, they cannot contribute'. Studying or doing research in moral philosophy does not bestow moral expertise. Philosophical medical ethics is not like engineering. When concrete real-life dilemmas are faced, philosophers, physicians, nurses and lay people are all on the same level – no one has special expertise over the others. Alternatively, as one of my own students suggested, if anyone has such 'expertise' then it must be the patient! They after all are the main actor in the play, and medicine would not exist without their problem and their suffering.

Even though they lack this 'moral expertise', philosophy and philosophers can still contribute to medical ethics in other important ways. Because medicine is so value-laden a discipline, there is plenty of work for philosophers in exploring the values that are to be found in various medical settings. Conceptual analysis is one of the tools of philosophers. If any discipline is full of vague concepts, surely it is medicine. Both philosophy and medicine can gain from this co-operation. Philosophical problems in medicine provide a real challenge to philosophy, which can in turn help to clarify the discussion.

References

Honderich T (ed.) (1995) *The Oxford Companion to Philosophy*. Oxford University Press, Oxford.

O'Neill O (1991) Introducing ethics: some current positions. *Bull Med Ethics*. **73**: 18–21.

Welie J (1998) *In the Face of Suffering. The philosophical–anthropological foundations of clinical ethics*. Creighton University Press, Omaha, NE.

'I'll just have another sit down for a minute, then I'm off home,' said the registrar to the ward manager. Now his entire left arm was aching. He still felt sick. He wondered about asking for some painkillers.

A trolley was wheeled into the room. Under the sheet lay an old man. A urinary catheter descended from the covers. The trolley stopped near the doctor's seat, and the old man cast a quizzical look at him.

'Just a part of getting old,' he said cheerfully. 'You never take peeing seriously until you can't do it any more.'

He looked at the doctor. 'What happened to you, my lad?'

'Well, I cut my thumb, pretty badly as it turns out. In the operating theatre of all places.'

'You were operating, then?'

'Yes, or trying to.'

'I was a doctor, too. I retired, oh, more than 20 years ago. Would you believe it,' he gestured towards the catheter, 'I was a urologist.' He chuckled. 'I spent more than 30 years of my life dealing with the problems of peeing, and I never once thought about how difficult life might get if you were the one who couldn't actually pass urine when you wanted to. And now I'm lying here with this drainpipe in my bladder.'

'So here we are, two doctors on the sick list – not much use to anyone else for a while. Ironic, isn't it?' He winced slightly and seemed to be in some discomfort. 'You know, the older you get in this game, the more you realise that medicine's not really about drugs, or silicon tubes, or defibrillators or any of the tools of the trade. And not just getting old. It's when you can't pee that you see that life is a mystery – a philosophical matter when you get down to it. If you deal with people's lives, you're in a philosophical business all the way. Oh, here comes *my* philosopher – I'm going to be seen to. Well, I hope that hand gets better soon. Cheerio!'

So is all this really relevant? My first 50 years in medical theory, practice and philosophy of medicine

Pekka Vuoria

A 62-year-old man was rushed to a university hospital emergency room with severe chest pain. A myocardial infarction (MI) was suspected, and appropriate measures were taken. However, the ECG showed no sign of MI, and the doctors decided to do some more tests to evaluate the patient's condition. The patient was given analgesics and the nurse took him to a side room to wait for the laboratory technician to draw some blood samples. The patient was perspiring and tired, and he kept his eyes closed as he tried to deal with the pain that was slowly subsiding.

The patient's wife came to the clinic to stay with her spouse. She asked a nurse about her husband's condition. Since the nurse was not in charge of the patient, she asked the wife to wait in a lobby. After half an hour or so the wife asked a cleaner where her husband was. The cleaner showed the woman to the patient's room.

The patient's chest pain was increasing again. His wife rang the bell and a nurse came in. The wife told the nurse that there had been aortic aneurysms in her husband's family, and suggested that this could be the cause of the patient's pain. The nurse promised to deliver this information to the doctor.

After a while a resident physician came in and the wife repeated the story about the aneurysms in the family. The doctor reassured her, saying that tests were on the way, and that she should not worry about anything – everything was under control. The resident left the couple alone. After an hour or so the laboratory technician came in and took blood samples. The patient was perspiring heavily and asked for some more analgesics. The technician promised to tell the nurse.

Another hour passed and a nurse came in. She gave the patient an injection to ease the pain, and she said they would take him to the X-ray department in a while, which they did.

After a further couple of hours the patient was brought back to the emergency room to wait for the results of the chest X-ray. His condition was getting worse. He felt extremely tired and the pain was excruciating. His wife went to look for a doctor. The work shift had changed, and she now found a junior resident who had not seen the patient before. The wife spoke about the possibility of aortic aneurysm and the doctor promised to consult a senior house officer about the problem.

An elderly doctor came in to evaluate the patient's condition. He told the nurse to bring an ultrasound device to the room. While they were installing the machine the patient died. An autopsy revealed that he had indeed died because of a ruptured aortic aneurysm.

This story is fictional, but incidents like these do happen.

Why? And what does this have to do with the philosophy of medicine?

In my later years – I am 78years of age at the time of writing – I have been contemplating the necessary conditions for good medical practice. Somewhere in my long career, starting as a country GP and retiring as a professor of radiology, I began to realise that the fundamental questions of medicine are not technical but philosophical in nature. When I use the word 'philosophical' here, I am referring to three aspects of medical theory and practice.

Medical practice considers and approaches the patient according to the prevailing theory of disease. This theory is in turn built on how we under- stand the notion of 'disease'. This constitutes what in philosophy is called *ontology* – that is, the basic orientations that we apply when we address the phenomena of the world – what general kinds of things we think there are to be found in the world, and how we will therefore classify them. In medicine we are concerned specifically with the ontology of disease.

The second aspect is closely related to the first one. If disease is defined in a particular way, what kind of knowledge is needed to explore and deal with disease, and how is that knowledge to be obtained? In philosophy the study of how we know things is called *epistemology*. In the general theory of medicine, epistemology asks (among other things) how we know about the general phenomena of disease. And within the practice of medicine it asks (among other things) how we know about this particular person's disease.

The third aspect – a fundamental (and philosophical) question in medicine – deals with the idea of good medical practice. Medicine addresses the wellbeing of the patient. This is a question of values. Why should we care about anyone's wellbeing? Why do we take care of our fellow beings in a state of pain and suffering? What constitutes their well-being or our 'taking care' of them? Thus, more generally, what constitutes sound medical practice? In philosophy these questions belong to the realm of moral philosophy or *ethics*. In medical practice we are increasingly involved with ethical problems that arise from the rapid development of medical technology. However, the question of ethical medical practice does not limit itself to the use of technology alone. It arises when encountering each and every individual patient with his or her specific problems and, more generally, from the way in which we ultimately finance and deliver medical service to the population as a whole.

Listen, look and remain silent

I started my career as a GP in a remote rural village in Eastern Finland in the 1950s. As a newly qualified physician, my approach to my patients was disease-centred. In those days, more often than not one saw patients suffering from such diseases as pulmonary tuberculosis, diphtheria, poliomyelitis, severe abscesses, pneumonias, etc. These diseases are now rare in Finland, owing to the improved standard of housing, schooling and nutrition as well as to extensive vaccination programmes. However, many if not most of those same conditions are still flourishing in many parts of the world – even just behind our Eastern border in Russian Karelia. (This lends support to the idea that diseases are not primarily medical problems but social and political issues, just as Rudolf Virchow, the founder of modern pathology, argued more than 100 years ago.)

I once made a house call to a family where an 18-year-old woman had been suffering from a high fever for several days. The girl was shy and quiet, and did not complain of any particular sign or symptom of any particular disease. The family was of no help to me. They just stood quietly and looked at me with their eyes full of respect for a doctor waiting to solve the problem of their daughter's illness.

I listened to the girl's lungs and heart, palpated her abdomen and looked into her throat. She was obviously running a high fever, but otherwise I could not find anything wrong with her. I then decided to act like a good physician, and I conducted a thorough medical examination by the book, from head to heels. I was more than happy to observe a flourishing infection deep in the skin of her left foot, even though the girl had not reported any problems in her leg. I gave her a series of injections with the then new wonder drug penicillin, and the girl was cured in no time. Besides gaining me a much needed good reputation among the villagers, this event reinforced my idea of what good medical practice is – I had better not give up until I find a reasonable explanation for the patient's problem.

However, a patient is not only an object of external evaluation. Many are the instances when I have gone astray merely by not paying proper attention to what the patient or her relatives have been telling me – or have been trying to tell me – because I have not listened or heard their stories properly.

Audi, vide, tace. Listen carefully, look and be silent. These are the traditional prerequisites of good doctoring. However, studies have shown that nowadays many doctors listen to their patient for less then 20 seconds before interrupting them – even though if the patient is given the chance to tell his or her story uninterrupted it will take only about 20 seconds more. Why is this so? If we as doctors do not offer our patients these precious moments we neglect the most important tool in our work – namely the patient's own account of his or her problem. And while doing this we also endanger or even lose the patient's trust, which is the prerequisite of all doctoring.

During the last couple of decades there has been growing interest in the doctor's communication skills. However, the way in which we approach our patients is not a matter of communication alone. This brings us back to the ontology of medicine. What is a patient?

If the patient is seen merely as a dysfunctioning organism, he will be studied with biological concepts and methods and treated accordingly. In this case communication may remain solely a question of good manners. However, if the patient is seen as a person approaching a doctor in order to find an explanation, alleviation, comfort and cure for his problems, the question of communication becomes a central issue in the whole medical endeavour. Furthermore, if we choose to define human illness by biochemical terms alone, we may develop approaches for classifying and treating those problems wholesale, addressing ourselves to classes of diseases instead of developing individual treatments for individual patients. The former calls for an 'industrial' approach to the delivery of medical care based on statistical guidelines, while the latter calls for personal physicians serving individuals.

Too often one hears of doctors who do not seem to care about their patients, considering their problems to be trivial and thus uninteresting. Perhaps such doctors are reluctant to enter into a personal encounter with their patients. They may, for example, just give the patient a prescription for paracetamol and send them away. In such a situation the patient's confidence may be lost – confidence which is, after all, one of the basic prerequisites of good medical care. As Francis Peabody, one of the central figures in early twentieth-century clinical medicine, once said: 'One of the essential qualities of the clinician is interest in humanity, for the secret of the care *of* the patient is in caring *for* the patient'.

Too many of the errors and poor results in medical care result from approaching the patient solely as a biological object. This may lead, in the worst cases, to indifference and neglect or even negligence – not caring about the patient as a person. By contrast, a good doctor is not negligent but instead tries persistently and tirelessly to evaluate the patient's signs, symptoms, fears and worries in order to understand what brought the patient to the surgery in the first place. To develop and cultivate this attitude to the patient is a necessary condition for being a good physician.

Nearly everything I have learned about medical practice I have learned from my patients – a great deal of it in general practice. I believe the same is more or less true for anyone in medical practice. The practising physician can learn from each and every patient if they only keep their mind open, and this will enable them to manage their patients well. It also offers them the best recompense anyone can get for a job done competently – a fulfilling sense of achievement when the patient gets well. If things go wrong and the patient does not improve or even dies, even then a physician can have a good conscience about having done their best for the patient.

'Act, but act at your peril'

Biomedical research gives medicine a rapidly expanding scientific basis. Developments in understanding the human genome, as well as knowledge of the cellular and metabolic bases of inflammatory and degenerative diseases, open up for us new possibilities with regard to understanding and treating major disease processes.

However,there is still the problem of how we should apply this expanding medical knowledge to medical practice. 'Evidence-based medicine' is an attempt to solve this problem. Yet every patient, and every clinical encounter between a patient and a doctor, is unique, and by definition there is not an evidence-based solution available for every medical situation. Therefore only by studying the patient's illness and progress towards recovery closely can doctors place themselves in a position to evaluate – together with the patient – whether their treatment is suitable for this particular patient in this particular episode of sickness.

But how can the doctor know what is right and what is wrong for the patient? The answer is that they cannot know with certainty. Let us consider a female patient who has a node in her breast (felt by palpation or seen at mammography). A needle biopsy is taken and it gives a negative result – that is, no malignant cells are found. This does not prove that there are no malignant cells in the breast. Perhaps the needle has not been inserted in the malignant part of the palpated node, or perhaps the radiologist has misinterpreted the X-ray finding.

Alternatively, let us consider the case of an elderly woman who died of viral pneumonia. Her chest X-ray is meticulously rechecked in a clinico-pathological meeting, but no abnormal signs indicating pneumonia can be seen. When I point this out in the meeting, the professor of pathology says that of course the viral pneumonic foci could not be seen on the X-ray because they were so small, and they could only be seen under a micro-scope after autopsy. A further example of this might arise in the case of tuberculosepsis. The patient has a general tuberculous infection causing high fever, but at the beginning of this fatal attack the foci in the lungs are too small to be seen on a normal radiographic film. In many other infectious conditions, such as mastitis, pyelonephritis, osteomyelitis and tonsillitis, the patient may have high fever, malaise and shivers but no local signs of the disease, which may not appear until 6 to 12 hours after the beginning of the general signs. High-quality biomedical data can elude us simply because many diseases cause changes that are not detectable by technical means in the preliminary phases of the disease. In such cases a proven method for clinical practice is to make recurrent re-examinations until the local signs appear and guide us to the correct diagnosis.

In 1929, John Dewey wrote that 'the distinctive characteristic of prac-tical activity, one which is so inherent that it cannot be eliminated, is the uncertainty which attends it. Of it we are compelled to say: act, but act at your peril.' A practical activity such as clinical medicine deals with indivi-dualised and unique situations and processes that are never exactly duplicable. Therefore no complete assurance is possible.

In medicine the randomised prospective double-blind clinical trial is considered to be the 'gold standard' of scientific research. However, this approach may easily fall into what I call a 'triple-blind study' if the selec-tion of patients under study is biased – as it sometimes is – in one way or another. A practising physician needs to be cautious when evaluating the significance of clinical trials for the care of his patients. If a double-blind study shows that the treatment studied is beneficial *and* the clinical evidence in the case in question supports this finding, then the treatment may be used with *some* degree of confidence. After all, the patient's overall response is a valuable (although, interestingly, not definitive) criterion for the success of the treatment that he or she receives.

In the service of the patient

Our society has a tendency to set up larger and larger organisations. This tendency is justified by calling it 'rationalising'. However, in medicine large organisations may have adverse effects with regard to its main task – taking care of the sick.

In medical practice the focal point is the encounter between the patient and the physician. This event is always non-repeatable, and it cannot therefore be standardised without losing its unique essence. If the organisation interferes with and aims to control the form and content of this encounter, then it reduces the autonomy of both the patient and the doctor, and it has a negative impact on the uniqueness of the individual doctor–patient relationship.

Large systems create parasitic functions. Healthcare organisations are increasingly used for purposes other than medical ones, that is, in pursuit of political, social, economical and personal interests. However we need to bear in mind that the primary aim of medical endeavour is taking care of the sick. This makes medicine essentially an *ethical* discipline. Building a healthcare system and setting priorities in it are therefore ethical issues. Too often, however, they are treated as if they were primarily economical, managerial or technological problems. Yet taking care of patients – and indeed the setting of priorities – ultimately happens at the bedside or in the surgery, where the clinical encounter takes place. Then – and only then – the knowledge, skills and abilities of the physician and the needs of the patient or their family can meet and bring cure and comfort to those in need.

It seems to me that the mega-systems of public medical care have a tendency to neglect the individual person and his or her personal features and needs. However, meeting an individual patient's needs is the primary reason for the existence of medicine in the first place. Modern systems are complex, and their flaws cannot be corrected by small measures. Perhaps the best and even the only method for bringing medicine back to its roots – that is, to the service of the patient – would be to give the patient the power to choose when, where and by whom he or she will be medically examined and, if necessary, treated.

The way in which we perceive our patients orientates us to the problems that they bring to our attention. Our basic orientations guide us not only in the way we as doctors address our patients, but also in the way we build, develop and maintain our healthcare system as a whole. Involvement for more than 50 years in medical practice, research, education and theory has deeply convinced me that philosophical reflection is not only relevant to medicine, but is the prerequisite of sound medical practice.

Reference

Dewey J (1929) *The Quest for Certainty: a study of the relation of knowledge and action.* Gifford Lectures. Minton, Balch & Co, New York.

The day ends

'You're home early, love. I didn't hear the car. God, what happened to your hand?'
'Oh, nothing. I just cut my left thumb.'

Index